Workbook with Lab Exercises
to Accompany
Principles of Radiographic Imaging
An Art and a Science

4th Edition

Workbook with Lab Exercises
to Accompany
Principles of Radiographic Imaging
An Art and a Science

4th Edition

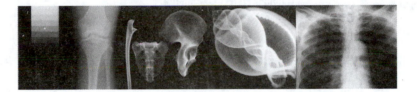

Revised by
Debra J. Poelhuis, MS, RT(R)(M)
Director, Radiography Program
Montgomery County Community College
Pottstown, Pennsylvania

Nina Kowalczyk, MS, RT(R)(CT)(QM), FASRT
Clinical Instructor
The Ohio State University
Columbus, Ohio

William F. Finney, III, MA, RT(R)
Acting Director and Assistant Professor
School of Allied Medical Professions
The Ohio State University
Columbus, Ohio

Richard R. Carlton, MS, RT(R)(CV), FAERS
Director, Radiologic and Imaging Sciences
Grand Valley State University
Grand Rapids, Michigan

Arlene M. Adler, MEd, RT(R), FAERS
Professor and Director, Radiologic Sciences Programs
Indiana University Northwest
Gary, Indiana

THOMSON

DELMAR LEARNING

Australia   Canada   Mexico   Singapore   Spain   United Kingdom   United States

THOMSON

DELMAR LEARNING

Workbook with Lab Exercises to Accompany Principles of Radiographic Imaging: An Art and a Science

by Rick R. Carlton and Arlene M. Adler

**Vice President,
Health Care Business Unit:**
William Brottmiller

Director of Learning Solutions:
Matthew Kane

Acquisitions Editor:
Maureen Rosener

Product Manager:
Laurie Traver

Senior Product Manager:
Darcy M. Scelsi

Editorial Assistant:
Elizabeth Howe

Marketing Director:
Jennifer McAvey

Marketing Channel Manager:
Tamara Caruso

Marketing Coordinator:
Chris Manion

Technology Director:
Laurie Davis

Technology Project Manager:
Mary Colleen Liburdi

Technology Project Coordinator:
Carolyn Fox

Production Director:
Carolyn Miller

Production Manager:
Barbara A. Bullock

Art and Design Coordinator:
Alexandros Vasilakos
Christi DiNinni

Production Coordinator:
Kenneth McGrath

Project Editor:
Jennifer Luck

NOTICE TO THE READER

Dedicated to

Abbie and Andy Poelhuis

William Leth

Nick and Doug Kowalczyk

Contents

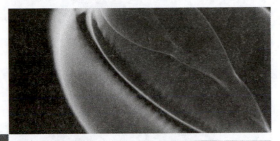

UNIT I   Creating the Beam

UNIT II   Protecting Patients and Personnel

UNIT III   Creating the Image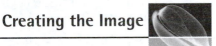

UNIT IV Analyzing the Image

UNIT V Comparing Exposure Systems

UNIT VI Special Imaging Systems

Preface

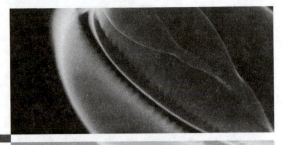

This workbook has been designed to correlate with the textbook *Principles of Radiographic Imaging: An Art and a Science,* 4th edition. Our intent has been to design a series of activities, both laboratories and worksheets, to provide higher level synthesis and analysis activities for each chapter in the textbook. There are 98 exercises, of which 68 are laboratories and 30 are worksheets. There is at least one exercise for each text chapter, with multiple activities for chapters that require exercises to assist students in understanding the more difficult concepts. Linear and semilog graph paper masters are included at the end of the workbook for use where applicable.

This workbook represents a correlated series of exercises to help strengthen didactic instruction. There are sufficient activities to support a regularly scheduled laboratory for courses in physics, principles of exposure, and imaging. An equipment chart is provided to assist faculty in preparing for each laboratory and for ordering supplies and equipment prior to each course.

Students are expected to be able to operate radiographic equipment, a film processor, densitometer, sensitometer, oscilloscope, and dosimeter for various exercises. No worksheets or laboratories are provided to teach students the operation of this equipment, since we found wide differ-

ences in manufacturers' operating instructions. We suggest that students be shown how to operate each new piece of equipment at the start of the laboratory where it must be used. Alternatively, faculty may produce laboratory exercises for this purpose by duplicating the relevant portions of the manufacturer's operating manual.

Many of the exercises in this workbook were based on laboratories that have been in use for many years at The Ohio State University, Lima Technical College, and Indiana University Northwest. A number of exercises were designed specifically for the chapters in the textbook. All of the activities were tested and found to be sound in concept. Additional testing was done by Barry Burns at the University of North Carolina. Each activity has a set of instructions with reasonable equipment requirements and preparation time.

We acknowledge responsibility for all errors in content. It is the responsibility of faculty to properly prepare students for laboratory coursework, and therefore we assume no responsibility for damage to equipment or persons as a result of students performing these exercises. In addition, information in this workbook should only be used in clinical practice subservient to prevailing procedures and under the direction of appropriate supervisory personnel.

Exposure Technique Factors

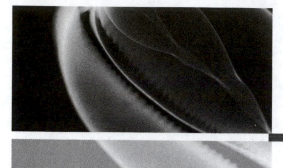

The use of these laboratories requires fine adjustment of exposure technical factors for each exercise. Most of the experiments that use radiographic film are based on the use of a 400 relative speed film/screen combination. Because of the complex variations in diagnostic imaging systems, it is impossible to suggest exposure factors that will produce ideal results in all situations. Faculty members may wish to produce the images for each experiment in order to obtain exact technical factors prior to assigning the laboratories to students.

Alternately, if students are working individually or in small groups, the entire group may learn valuable lessons by assisting in adjusting our suggested factors until an ideal density has been achieved for each activity. In all cases, the **image density should be adjusted by mAs changes only** (unless otherwise stated in the laboratory instructions). **Kilovoltage levels have been chosen for specific effects in many experiments and should not be changed unless absolutely necessary due to equipment limitations.**

Laboratory Equipment and Materials

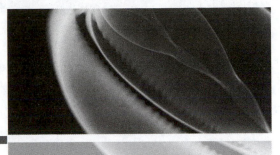

The majority of laboratory activities contained in this manual require specific items that are common to a radiography environment. In order to facilitate the instructor and student in preparing for the laboratory activities, the following equipment/materials matrix lists the basic equipment and material requirements for each laboratory experiment. For a more complete description of the recommended items, the reader should refer to the specific laboratory experiment. Laboratories listed with a # sign indicate items with alternative choices or options for completion of the experiment. Those listed with a * sign indicate that the items have to be prepared or constructed prior to the experiment. Refer to the specific experiment for detailed instructions. Keep in mind that the equipment/materials recommendations have been made based on field trials and are not etched in stone, so feel free to substitute the equipment and/or material items if deemed necessary. Remember that ingenuity is the mother of all experiments.

3-1	**3-2**	**4-1**	**4-2**
Electroscope	1.5 V battery (5) or DC power source	#9 V battery (dry cell)	Bar magnets (different strengths)
Static rods	Ammeter/Voltmeter	Bar magnets	Galvanometer or ammeter
Silk patches	Copper wire	Cardboard, stiff paper, plexiglass (8 × 10)	*Wire helix coils
Wool patches	Resistors (Five 5-watt)	Compass	Copper wire with alligator clips
		Galvanometer or ammeter	
		Iron filings	
		Wire (3′)	

5-2	**6-1**	**8-1**	**9-1**
Cable/BNC connectors	X-ray tube parts	Dosimeter	Dosimeter
Radiographic unit		Phantom body part	Gonad shields
Storage oscilloscope		Radiographic unit	Phantom body part
X-ray output detector		Ring stand	Radiographic unit
			Ring stand

10-1

0.25, 0.5, 1.0, 2.0 mm
  Al filters
Radiographic unit
Dosimeter

10-2

Radiographic unit
Four 1 mm Al
  attenuators
Dosimeter

11-2

Dosimeter
Radiographic unit

13-1

Digital dosimeter
Radiographic unit
Technique chart

14-1

Cassette/image
  receptor
Dosimeter
Film processor
Phantom body part
Radiographic unit

15-1

Cassette/image
  receptor
Film processor
Phantom body part
Plastic gallon jugs
Radiographic unit
CR cassette or DR

16-1

Cassette/imge receptor
Cassette holder
Dosimeter
Film processor
Phantom body part
Radiographic unit
Wire mesh tool

17-1

Teaching radiographs

18-1

Aluminum step wedge
Cassette/image
  receptor
Densitometer
Film processor
Phantom body part
8:1 and 12:1 grids
Radiographic unit

18-2

Cassette/image
  receptor
Film processor
Phantom body part
12:1 grid
Radiographic unit

18-3

Cassette/image
  receptor
Densitometer
Film processor
Phantom body part
Radiographic unit

18-4

Radiographic Unit
Cassettes (2)
Phantom
8:1 and 12:1 grids (2)

19-4

Cassette/image
  receptor
Film processor
Hand lotion

19-5

Densitometer
Duplication film
Duplication unit
Film processor
Radiograph, good
  quality
Radiograph,
  overexposed

20-2

Densitometer
Film processor
Radiographic image
  receptor
Sensitometer
Thermometer

20-3

Film processor

21-1

Densitometer
Film processor
Graph paper
3 types of radiographic
  orthochromatic film
Sensitometer

22-1

Aluminum step wedge
Densitometer
Film processor
Radiographic unit
2 blue light-emitting
  rare-earth cassettes
  with different RS
  values
2 green light-emitting
  rare-earth cassettes
  with different RS
  values

23-1

Aluminum step wedge
Cassettes/image
  receptors (variety)
Densitometer
Dosimeter
Film processor
Phantom body part
Radiographic unit
Resolution test tool

24-2

CT unit
MRI unit

25-1
Cassette/image
  receptor
CR imaging system
Film processor
Phantom body part

25-2
Radiographic unit
5 CR cassettes
Screen/film cassette
Phantom body part
Film processor

27-1
Radiographic unit
Phantom body part
Cassette
CR cassettes or DR unit
  film processor
CR image processor
Film processor

28-1
Aluminum step wedge
Cassette/image
  receptor
Densitometer
Film processor
Phantom body part
Radiographic unit

28-2
Aluminum step wedge
Cassette/image
  receptor
Densitometer
Film processor
Phantom body part
Radiographic unit

28-3
Cassette/image
  receptor
Densitometer
Film processor
Phantom body part
Radiographic unit
CR image processor
CR cassettes

28-4
Aluminum step wedge
Cassette/image
  receptor
Densitometer
Film processor
Phantom body part
Radiographic unit

28-5
Aluminum step wedge
Densitometer
Film processor
Phantom body part
Radiographic unit
Various speed cassettes
  with image receptor

28-6
1″ Super ball
35 mm film canister
Barium solution
3″ to 4″ container
Cassettes/image
  receptor
Film processor
Ice cubes
Radiographic unit
Note: These films are
  also used for
  Laboratory 29-3

29-1
Aluminum step wedge
Cassette/image
  receptor
Densitometer
Film processor
Phantom body part
Radiographic unit

29-2
Aluminum step wedge
Densitometer
Film processor
Radiographic unit
Various speed cassettes
  with image receptor

29-3
Use films/supplies from
  28-6

29-4
Cassette/image
  receptor
Film processor
Phantom body part
Radiographic unit

29-5
Aluminum step wedge
Cassette/image
  receptor
Densitometer
Film processor
Phantom body part
Radiographic grids
Radiographic unit

30-1
Cassette/image
  receptor
Dry bones
Film processor
Radiographic unit
Resolution test pattern
Sponges
Lead masks

30-2
Cassette/image
  receptor
Dry bones
Film processor
Radiographic unit
Resolution test pattern
Sponges

30-3
Film processor
Phantom body part
Radiographic unit
Resolution test pattern
Sponge
Various speed cassettes
  with image receptor

30-4
Nonscreen film
  holder/image
  receptor
Film processor
Phantom body part
Radiographic unit
String

31-1
Cassette/image
  receptor
Small dry bone
  (vertebrae preferred)
Film processor
Metric ruler
Radiographic unit

31-2
Cassette/image
  receptors
Dry bones
Film processor
Metric ruler
Radiographic unit

32-1

Repeated images

33-1

Densitometer
Film processor
Sensitometer
Radiographic film
Thermometer

33-2

Nonscreen film
  holder/film
Film processor
Metric ruler
Radiographic unit
Star test pattern

33-3

Beam perpendicularity
  test tool
Cassettes/image
  receptors
#Collimator test tool
Film processor
Nine pennies
Radiographic unit with
  PBL
Scrap film
Paper clips

33-4

Cassette/image
  receptor
Film processor
Metric ruler
Radiographic unit
Ring stand
Scrap film
Bubble level
Angulator
Quarter or other coin

33-5

#Densitometer
Digital kVp meter
Film processor
#kVp test cassette
  (with current
  calibration chart)
Radiographic unit

33-6

Cassette/image
  receptor
Film processor
Motorized
  synchronous top
Protractor
Radiographic unit
Digital exposure timer

33-7

Digital dosimeter
Radiographic unit

33-8

Adhesive tape
Cassettes, empty
Cassette/image
  receptor
Film processor
Gauze pads
Radiographic unit
Screen cleaner
Wire mesh test tool

33-9

Light meter
View boxes
View box test template

33-10

Repeated images
Repeat analysis
  worksheet

33-11

Cardboard
Cassette/image
  receptor
Film processor
Radiographic unit
Densitometer

35-1

Cassette/image
  receptor
Film processor
Phantom body part
Radiographic unit

36-1

Cassette/image
  receptor
Film processor
Phantom body part
Radiographic unit

37-1

Cassette/image
  receptor
Film processor
Phantom body part
Radiographic unit with
  ion chamber AEC

37-2

Cassette/image
  receptor
Film processor
Phantom body part
Radiographic unit with
  AEC

37-3

Cassette/image
  receptor
Film processor
Lead masking
Phantom body part
Radiographic unit with
  AEC

37-4

3/4″ Aluminum plates
Cassette/imge receptor
Densitometer
Film processor
Lead markers
Radiographic unit
  with AEC

39-1

Cassette/image
  receptor
Film processor
Coconut
Radiographic unit

40-1

Cassette/image
  receptor
Film processor
Fluoroscopic unit
Lead apron
Phantom body part

40-2

Cassette/image
  receptor
Film processor
Fluoroscopic unit
Lead apron
Phantom body part

41-2

Cassette/image
  receptor
Film processor
Tomographic unit
Tomographic test
  phantom

45-2

CT images, abdomen
MRI images, abdomen

Creating the Beam

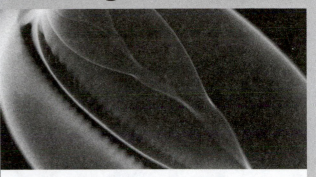

WORKSHEET 1–1 BASIC MATHEMATICS REVIEW

PURPOSE

Drill and practice in solving basic mathematical problems.

FOR FURTHER REVIEW

Refer to Chapter 1 in the accompanying textbook for further review of this topic.

ACTIVITIES

Carry out the math operations indicated and solve the following problems:

Problems for Fractions

1. $1/9 + 4/9 =$

2. $4/9 - 2/9 =$

3. $2/5 \div 3/4 =$

4. $3/4 \cdot 1/5 =$

5. $2/3 \div 5/7 =$

Problems for Decimals

1. $(34.21) \cdot (1.1) =$

2. $714.58 + 214.785 =$

3. $725 \div 0.25 =$

4. Change 85% to a decimal.

5. Change 0.081 to a percent.

Problems for Computation with Values (Numbers)

1. Round each of the following to the number of significant digits indicated.

   a. 328.14 (4)

   b. 1.25 (2)

   c. 2,709 (3)

2. Multiply or divide the following numbers, leaving the result with the correct number of significant digits if each number is assumed to be approximate.

   a. (2.32)(1.2)

   b. (43.81) ÷ (2.23)

3. Multiply or divide the following numbers, leaving the result with the correct number of significant digits if each number is assumed to be approximate.

   a. (38.42)(3.82)

   b. (4.32) ÷ (1.5)

4. Add or subtract the following numbers, leaving the result with the correct number of significant digits if each number is assumed to be approximate.

   a. 21.3 + 21.39

   b. 48.61 + 61

5. How many significant digits are in each of the following?

a. 7.04

b. 180

c. 180.0

d. 9,300

e. 8104.6

Problems for Scientific Notation

1. Change the following numbers to scientific notation.

a. 784.2

b. 0.00431

c. 78,210,000

d. 0.0000067

e. 7.4

2. Change the following numbers to ordinary notation.

a. 2.84×10^5

b. 2.84×10^{-5}

c. 6.18×10^0

d. 6.18×10^{-2}

e. 6.18×10^1

Problems for Signed Numbers

1. $(-6) - (-9) + (-6) =$

2. $(-8)(-2)(-3) =$

3. $(15) \div (-13) =$

4. $-6 - 8 - 2 + 3 =$

5. $(-2)(-1)(-1)(-1) =$

Problems for Order of Operation

1. Evaluate each of the following:

a. $17 - 8.2 + 4 \cdot 5 - 2.6^2$

b. $(3 + 1)^2 - 4(8 + 2) - 5 \cdot (-1)$

c. $6(2^2 - 4 \cdot 1) - 4^2$

d. $-2(3 + 4 \cdot 5)$

e. $(-8)^2 + 3 \cdot 5^2$

2. Evaluate each of the following:

a. $7 + 4 \cdot 5$

b. $6 \cdot 7 - 4 \cdot (-6)$

c. $2 \cdot 7^2$

d. $(-4)^2$

e. -4^2

f. $6(7 + 3) + 4 \cdot 8 - 7^2$

Problems for Algebraic Expressions

1. Simplify the following algebraic expressions.

   a. $2(3x + 4y) + (x - y)$

   b. $2(x - 4y) - 6(x + 2y)$

   c. $6[2x - 4(x - y)]$

   d. $-3[2(x + 5y) - 6(2x + 3y)]$

2. Simplify the following algebraic expressions.

   a. $2(3x + 4y) + (x - y)$

   b. $3(x - 2y) - 6(x + y)$

   c. $4[3x - 2(2x - 3y)]$

   d. $8[-2(2x + 3) + 4(x - y)]$

Problems for Exponents

1. Simplify each of the following expressions, leaving the answer with only positive exponents.

   a. $a^4 \cdot a^5 \cdot a^3$

   b. $\dfrac{b^8 \cdot b^4}{b^5}$

   c. $(a^2)^3 (b^{-2})^{-5}$

   d. $\dfrac{a^4 b^2 a^8 b^6}{a^5 b^3 a^{10} b^2}$

2. Simplify each of the following expressions leaving the answer with only positive exponents.

   a. $a^2 \cdot a^4 \cdot a^8$

   b. $\dfrac{b^6 b^2}{b^5}$

   c. $a^2 \cdot b^5 \cdot a^5 \cdot b^2$

   d. $\dfrac{a^8 b^{10}}{a^{11} b^4}$

Problems for Evaluating Algebraic Expressions

1. Evaluate each of the following expressions for $a = 5$, $b = 3$, and $c = -2$.

   a. $a + b \cdot c$

   b. $a + b - c$

   c. $2c + 3b^2 + 2(a - c)$

2. Evaluate each of the following expressions for $a = 2$, $b = -4$, and $c = 6$.

   a. $2a + 3b - 4c$

   b. $b^2 - 2c^2 + a^2$

   c. $5(a + 2b - c) + 4 \cdot b$

Problems for Equations

1. Solve for x: $x/6 = 3$

2. Solve for y: $2y + 3 = 9$

3. Solve for b: $2(b + 6) = b + 12$

4. Solve for x: $18/11 = 3/x$

5. Solve for a: $3(a + 4) = 15$

WORKSHEET 1–2 UNITS OF MEASUREMENT

PURPOSE

Drill and practice in solving units of measurement and dimensional analysis problems.

FOR FURTHER REVIEW

Refer to Chapter 1 in the accompanying textbook for further review of this topic.

ACTIVITIES

Carry out the math operations indicated and solve the following problems:

Problems for Dimensional Analysis

Convert the following:

1. 15 inches to yards

2. 1,500 seconds to hours

3. 1.8 hours to seconds

4. 18.9 feet to inches

5. 60 miles/hour to feet/second

6. 44 feet/second to miles/hour

7. 10 feet^2 to inches^2

8. 10 meters^2 to centimeters^2

9. 14 inches^3 to feet^3

10. 15 yards^3 to feet^3

11. 15.8 g/cm^3 to kg/m^3

12. 6.8 gallons to pints

WORKSHEET 1-2 (Continued)

Identify the SI unit of measurement and symbol for the following quantities:

Quantity	Unit	Symbol
13. Length	_____	_____
14. Mass	_____	_____
15. Time	_____	_____
16. Exposure	_____	_____
17. Absorbed Dose	_____	_____
18. Dose Equivalent	_____	_____

Convert the following:

19. 500 milliroentgens to coulombs/kilogram

20. 20 millirem to sieverts

21. 50 rads to grays

22. 6.45×10^{-4} coulombs/kilogram to roentgens

23. 0.084 sievert to rems

24. 0.35 gray to rads

WORKSHEET 2-1 BASIC ATOMIC THEORY

PURPOSE

Describe the basic theory of atomic structure.

FOR FURTHER REVIEW

Refer to Chapter 2 in the accompanying textbook for further review of this topic.

ACTIVITIES

1. How do atoms differ from molecules? elements from compounds?

2. List the three basic subatomic particles along with their corresponding mass number and charge.

3. What is the difference between a neutral atom and an ion?

4. How is the identity of an element determined?

5. What is the difference among atomic number, mass number, and atomic weight?

6. Draw a diagram of an aluminum atom.

7. How many valence electrons does aluminum have?

8. Name two elements that have a single valence electron.

9. Identify the number of orbital shells for each of the following atoms:

   a. helium

   b. lead

   c. barium

   d. calcium

   e. oxygen

10. What is the maximum number of electrons that can occupy the K shell? L shell? M shell? N shell? O shell? P shell? Q shell?

11. Explain the octet rule.

12. What do all of the elements in Group 1 of the periodic table have in common?

13. What is the difference between an ionic bond and a covalent bond?

14. Draw a diagram of a water molecule.

WORKSHEET 2-2 ELECTROMAGNETIC RADIATION

PURPOSE

Identify and describe electromagnetic radiation and qualitatively and quantitatively demonstrate the relationships among wavelength, frequency, velocity, and energy.

FOR FURTHER REVIEW

Refer to Chapter 2 in the accompanying textbook for further review of this topic.

ACTIVITIES

Answer the following questions and solve the problems showing your calculations:

1. Rank in order the following types of electromagnetic radiation according to their wavelength, using #1 for the one with the longest wavelength and #8 for the one with the shortest wavelength.

   _____ visible light   _____ radiowaves

   _____ x-rays   _____ microwaves

   _____ ultraviolet light   _____ cosmic rays

   _____ gamma rays   _____ infrared light

2. Briefly describe what is meant by the wave-particle duality of radiation.

3. Describe the relationship among the frequency, wavelength, and velocity of an electromagnetic wave.

4. Describe the relationship among electromagnetic photon energy and its frequency.

5. Calculate the frequency of ultraviolet-blue light, which has a wavelength of 350 nanometers.

6. Calculate the frequency of a 1.77 Angstrom x-ray photon.

7. A popular FM radio station broadcasts at 100 MHz. Calculate the wavelength of this frequency.

8. Calculate the wavelength in nanometers of green light that has a frequency of 5×10^{14} Hz.

9. Calculate the energy in keV of an x-ray photon that has a frequency of 1.69×10^{19} Hz.

10. Calculate the energy in keV of an x-ray photon that has a wavelength of 0.05 nm.

LABORATORY 3-1 LAWS OF ELECTROSTATICS AND ELECTRODYNAMICS

PURPOSE

Interpret the results of various electrostatic interactions.

FOR FURTHER REVIEW

Refer to Chapter 3 in the accompanying textbook for further review of this topic.

MATERIALS

1. Electroscope

2. Static conducting rods or plastic strips

3. Small pieces of wool and silk

PROCEDURES

1. Always ground the electroscope by gently touching the knob with the palm of your hand prior to performing any experiment. If your electroscope has thin metal leaves, never touch them.

2. Use a piece of cloth to rub your conducting strip, then touch the knob of the electroscope. Record your observations. Repeat for each type of cloth available.

3. Use a piece of cloth to rub your conducting strip, then bring the conducting strip close to, but do not allow it to touch, the knob of the electroscope. Record your observations. Repeat for each type of cloth available.

RESULTS

1. Record the reaction that was observed in the electroscope for each type of cloth when the conducting rod or strip touched the knob.

2. Record the reaction that was observed in the electroscope for each type of cloth when the conducting rod or strip came near, but did not touch, the knob.

LABORATORY 3-1 (Continued)

ANALYSIS

Use two signs to indicate the presence of electrons. Do not use any + signs.

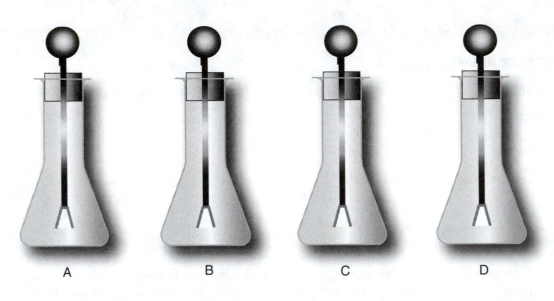

A   B   C   D

1. Use Figure A to indicate the distribution of electrons and the position of the leaves while a charged conducting rod was in contact with the knob.

2. Use Figure B to indicate the distribution of electrons and the position of the leaves after a charged rod was removed from contact with the knob.

3. Use Figure C to indicate the distribution of electrons and the position of the leaves while a charged rod was near, but not touching, the knob.

4. Use Figure D to indicate the distribution of electrons and the position of the leaves after a charged rod was removed from proximity with the knob.

5. Were there any differences in the effect seen with the various cloths? Why?

6. Which law of electrostatics was demonstrated in Figure A?

7. What is the term for the effect seen in Figure B?

8. What effect would be seen if the electroscope was subjected to an intense dose of ionizing radiation?

LABORATORY 3-2 OHM'S LAW AND RESISTANCE

PURPOSE

Demonstrate the relationships involved in Ohm's law.

FOR FURTHER REVIEW

Refer to Chapter 3 in the accompanying textbook for further review of this topic.

MATERIALS

1. DC variable power source (five 1.5-volt C or D size batteries can be substituted)

2. Five 10 Ω, 5-watt resistors

3. Meters capable of measuring 0 to 10 V and 0 to 1,000 mA (0 – 1 A)

4. Connecting wires

PROCEDURES

Effect of EMF on Current Flow

1. Connect two 10 Ω resistors in series and hook the combination in series with an ammeter and the power source. Use a voltmeter across the power source to set it at 1.5 V. Record the applied voltage and the current flow as measured by the ammeter (in the range of 75 mA).

2. Repeat step 1 four more times after increasing the voltage in increments of 1.5 volts up to a total of 7.5 volts while leaving the resistance the same.

Effect of Resistance on Current Flow

1. Use a voltmeter connected across the power source to adjust it to 6 V. Connect one 10 Ω resistor in series with the ammeter and hook the combination in series with the power source. Record the current measured by the ammeter (in the range of 600 mA).

2. Repeat step 1 for resistance values of 20, 30, 40, and 50 Ω by connecting in turn two, three, four, and five of the 10 Ω resistors in series.

LABORATORY 3-2 (Continued)

RESULTS

Effect of Voltage on Current Flow

1. Plot the following graph of current (I) against applied voltage (V) using the data obtained from steps 1 and 2. (Mark the vertical axis with mA values that will permit all your data to be graphed.)

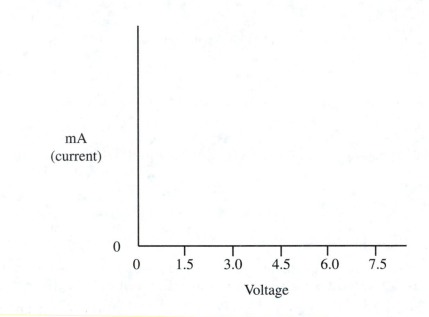

Effect of Resistance on Current Flow

1. Plot the following graph of current (I) against resistance (R) voltage using the data obtained from steps 1 and 2. (Mark the vertical axis with mA values that will permit all your data to be graphed.)

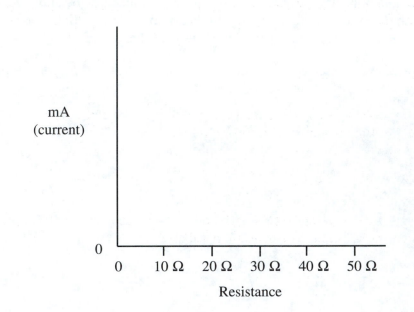

LABORATORY 3-2 (Continued)

ANALYSIS

Ohm's Law
Use Ohm's law to fill in the missing quantities in the chart.

	amps	volts	ohms
1.	100	_____	4
2.	56	_____	312
3.	_____	110	60
4.	_____	2,110	11.5
5.	50	110	_____
6.	0.8	39	_____

Effect of Series and Parallel Circuits on Resistance, Current, and EMF

7. What is the total resistance of a circuit if it contains resistances of 3 Ω, 2 Ω, and 10 Ω in series? in parallel?

8. What is the total resistance of a circuit if it contains resistances of 110 Ω, 26.2 Ω, and 14 Ω in series? in parallel?

9. If a circuit has resistances of 10 Ω, 12 Ω, and 2.4 Ω and an emf of 140 volts, what is the current if the circuit has the resistances in series? in parallel?

10. If a circuit has resistances of 10 Ω, 4.2 Ω, and 3 Ω and a current of 56 amps, what is the emf if the circuit has the resistances in series? in parallel?

Effect of Voltage on Current Flow

11. Based on the results of the experiment as shown on graph 1, when the resistance was relatively constant, what effect did voltage have on amperage? Is this finding consistent with Ohm's law?

Effect of Resistance on Current Flow

12. Based on the results of the experiment as shown on graph 2, when the voltage was relatively constant, what effect did resistance have on amperage? Is this finding consistent with Ohm's law?

LABORATORY 4-1 LAWS OF MAGNETISM AND MAGNETIC INDUCTION

PURPOSE

Demonstrate basic laws of magnetism, map static, and dynamic field flux lines, and illustrate the basic principle of magnetic induction.

FOR FURTHER REVIEW

Refer to Chapters 3 and 4 in the accompanying textbook for further review of this topic.

MATERIALS

1. Two bar magnets

2. Three pieces of stiff paper, cardboard, or Plexiglas (approximately 8″ × 10″)

3. Iron filings

4. 3′ length of wire

5. Low-voltage power supply or dry cell (about 9 V)

6. Compass

7. Galvanometer (or ammeter)

PROCEDURES

Laws of Magnetism

1. Place the two bar magnets end-to-end with both S poles about 3" apart. Hold both magnets tightly and bring the two ends together.

2. Repeat step 1 with a N and S pole together.

3. Repeat step 2 but hold the magnets away from each other at a distance of 2", 1", 1/2" while feeling the force of the magnetic field at each distance. Record the distances in order of magnetic field strength.

Mapping a Static Field

1. Level the paper with spacers to permit the bar magnet to be positioned underneath.

2. Sprinkle the iron filings on the paper over the magnet.

Mapping a Dynamic Field

3. Run a wire vertically through a hole in the center of the paper (as shown in the figure). Connect the ends of a low-voltage battery (9-volt dry cell suggested).

4. Draw arrows on the paper to map the direction of a compass needle (as shown in the textbook Figure 4-6). Place the compass on the surface of the paper and draw an arrow representing the direction of the compass needle. Slowly move the compass in a circle around the wire, adding arrows as the compass needle changes direction.

5. Reverse the connections of the wire at the battery and repeat step 4.

LABORATORY 4-1 (Continued)

Magnetic Induction

6. Connect a wire (or wire coil) to an ammeter. Wave a bar magnet close to, but not touching, the wire while observing the meter.

ANALYSIS

Laws of Magnetism

1. Which law of magnetism was illustrated by steps 1 and 2?

2. Which law of magnetism was illustrated by step 3?

3. State the law of magnetism that would require breaking the bar magnets.

Mapping a Static Field

4. Draw the configuration of the magnetic lines of flux as revealed by the iron filings.

5. Why do the iron filings represent the magnetic lines of force?

Mapping a Dynamic Field

6. What is represented by the changing of the direction of the compass needle?

7. Explain the reason for the change in the direction of the lines of force between steps 4 and 5.

8. Which of the Fleming hand rules is demonstrated by this experiment?

9. Draw in the appropriate compass needle directions, lines of force directions, and electron flow on Figure A for one direction flow and on Figure B for the other direction.

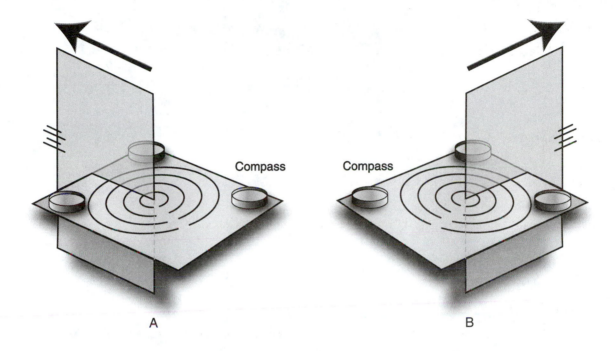

Compass   Compass

A   B

Magnetic Induction

10. What effect does a moving magnetic field have on the current in a wire (or coil of wire)?

11. Explain (at the atomic level) how a moving magnetic field causes electrons to move along a wire, thus producing current through magnetic induction.

12. Add arrows in the appropriate direction for the induced magnetic field in the following Figure C.

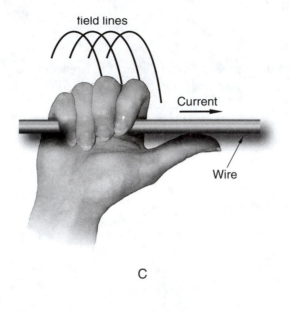

C

LABORATORY 4-2 ELECTROMAGNETIC INDUCTION

PURPOSE

Illustrate Faraday's Laws of electromagnetics.

FOR FURTHER REVIEW

Refer to Chapter 4 in the accompanying textbook for further review of this topic.

MATERIALS

1. Helix coil of wire with few turns
2. Helix coil of wire with many turns
3. Moderately strong bar magnet
4. Strong bar magnet
5. Galvanometer (or ammeter)
6. Two connecting wires (preferably with alligator clips)

PROCEDURES

1. Use the wires to connect the ends of the helix coil with few turns to the meter. Record the approximate meter reading when the moderately strong bar magnet is moved at an average speed inside the coil. (If the coil is too small to accommodate the magnet, the magnet may be used to "stroke" the outside of the coil without touching the wires.)

2. Repeat step 1 with the strong bar magnet.

3. Repeat step 2 at high, moderate, and slow speed.

4. Repeat step 2 but with the magnet outside the coil moving at a 90° angle to the wire coils. Record the approximate meter reading at 90°, 45°, and parallel to the wire coils.

5. Repeat step 2 using the coil with few turns and again using the coil with many turns.

ANALYSIS

1. Complete the following data chart:

AMPERE READINGS										
Strength		Speed			Angle			Number of turns	
moderate	strong	slow	moderate	high	90°	45°	0°	few	many

2. Which of Faraday's laws is demonstrated by procedure steps 1 and 2?

3. Which of Faraday's laws is demonstrated by procedure step 3?

4. Which of Faraday's laws is demonstrated by procedure step 4?

5. Which of Faraday's laws is demonstrated by procedure step 5?

6. Label the arrows on the following figure to illustrate which indicates the direction of the magnetic field, current, and motion.

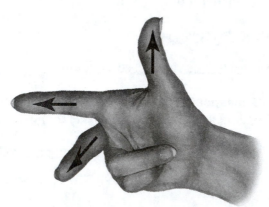

WORKSHEET 4–3 GENERATORS, MOTORS, AND ALTERNATING AND DIRECT CURRENT

PURPOSE

Explain the theory of generators and motors.

FOR FURTHER REVIEW

Refer to Chapters 3 and 4 in the accompanying textbook for further review of this topic.

ACTIVITIES

1. An electric generator converts _____ energy into _____ energy.

2. In a generator, the conducting loops across which an emf is induced are called the _____.

3. A current that moves in one direction during part of the generating cycle and in an opposite direction during the remainder of the cycle is a(n) _____.

4. The output of a generator is increased by increasing the _____, or by increasing the number of _____ on the armature.

5. In using Fleming's left-hand generator rule, when the thumb points in the direction the armature is moving and the index finger points in the direction of the magnetic flux, the middle finger indicates the direction of _____ flow.

6. A generator can supply _____ current if its armature turns are connected to a commutator.

7. An electric motor converts _____ energy into _____ energy.

8. In using Fleming's left-hand motor rule, when the thumb points in the direction the conductor is moving and the index finger points in the direction of the magnetic flux, the middle finger indicates the direction of _____ flow.

9. The synchronous motor is a constant _____ motor.

10. An induction motor uses a _____ to turn the rotor.

11. X-ray tubes use _____ motors to rotate the anode.

12. What are the essential components of an electric generator?

13. What are the essential components of an induction motor?

14. The following illustration represents the emf produced by an AC generator at various points as the armature coil wire rotates in the magnetic field.

    a. Draw arrows to show the direction of movement of the armature coil wire.

    b. Show conventional current flow through the armature coil wire at each point (A through I) in its rotation using the following method:

        1. Place a dot in the center of the conductor if the current flow is out of the page.
        2. Place a plus in the center of the conductor if the current flow is into the page.
        3. Leave the conductor blank if there is no current flow.

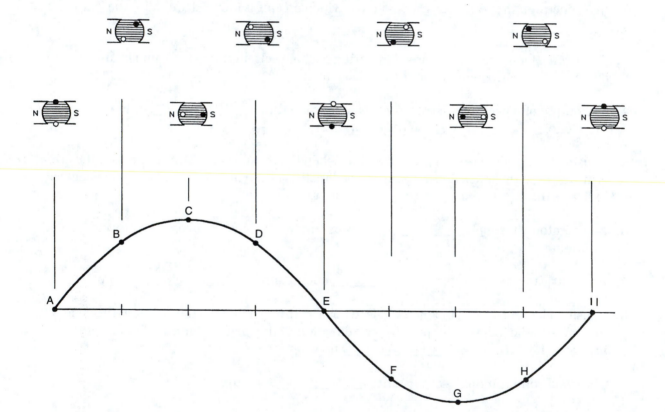

WORKSHEET 4-4 TRANSFORMERS, AUTOTRANSFORMERS, AND CAPACITORS

PURPOSE

Explain the effects of various types of transformers and capacitors on electrical current.

FOR FURTHER REVIEW

Refer to Chapter 4 in the accompanying textbook for further review of this topic.

ACTIVITIES

1. Explain the basic concept of how a transformer uses induction to transform current.

2. Why won't a transformer function when supplied with direct current?

3. Explain in detail two of the three primary causes of transformer power loss.

4. What is the primary difference between a transformer and an autotransformer?

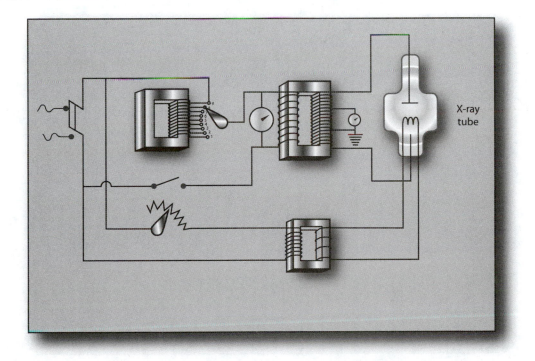

5. Label each transformer in the preceding drawing according to type (i.e., step-up, step-down, autotransformer). Place a "P" on the primary side and an "S" on the secondary side.

6. If a transformer is supplied with 200 volts to the primary coil, has 200 turns of wire on the primary coil and 40,000 turns of wire on the secondary coil, what will the voltage be in the secondary coil?

7. If a transformer has 1,600 turns of wire on the primary coil, 110 volts in the primary coil, and 10 volts in the secondary coil, how many turns of wire must there be in the secondary coil?

8. How does a capacitor function?

WORKSHEET 4–5 RECTIFICATION

PURPOSE

Analyze the direction of current flow for various rectification circuits.

FOR FURTHER REVIEW

Refer to Chapter 4 in the accompanying textbook for further review of this topic.

ACTIVITIES

1. In the space above, draw a simple half-wave rectification circuit in which a single diode is used to protect the x-ray tube.

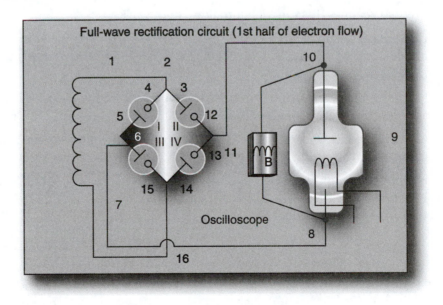

This figure may be replaced by an x-ray circuit simulator if one is available.

2. Observe the direction of the current at arrow 16 in the drawing. Draw in the appropriate arrows for 15 through 1 to show the direction of current for a full-wave rectification circuit.

3. Explain why the diode is placed on the cathode or anode side of a half-wave rectification circuit.

4. Number each of these descriptions to match the arrow in the drawing for #2.

_____   Conventional current flow is induced from the secondary coil of the high-voltage step-up transformer.

_____   Current on this path reaches the heated cathode of valve tube III and easily jumps to the anode (thus never permitting enough charge to accumulate for the current at arrow 14 to jump across valve tube IV).

_____   Current on this path reaches the anode of valve tube I and distributes over the large unheated surface, attempting to build up enough charge to jump to the cathode.

_____   Current on this path reaches the anode of valve tube IV and distributes over the large unheated surface, attempting to build up enough charge to jump to the cathode.

_____   Current on this path moves without resistance toward the x-ray tube.

_____   Current reaches the x-ray tube heated cathode and jumps to the anode.

_____   Current on this path reaches the heated cathode of valve tube IV but cannot jump to the anode because the anode is still loaded with the charge moving at arrow 14. Because these are like charges, they repel one another.

_____   X-rays are produced as a result of the current striking the anode.

_____   Current from the anode moves without resistance back toward the rectification circuit.

_____   Current reaches this junction and flows both ways.

_____   Current on this path reaches the heated cathode of valve tube II and easily jumps to the anode.

_____   Current reaches this junction and flows both ways.

_____   Current reaches this junction and flows both ways.

_____   Current on this path reaches the heated cathode of valve tube I but cannot jump to the anode because the anode is still loaded with the charge moving at arrow 5. Because these are like charges, they repel one another.

_____   From this point on, current on this path moves without resistance toward the secondary coil of the high-voltage step-up transformer.

_____   Current reaches the secondary coil of the high-voltage step-up transformer, completing the circuit.

5. Would current flow through the x-ray tube, and, if so, would it be full- or half-wave rectified if valve tube I burned out? II? III? IV?

6. Would current flow through the x-ray tube, and, if so, would it be full- or half-wave rectified if valve tubes I and II burned out? I and III? I and IV? II and III? II and IV? III and IV?

7. Would current flow through the x-ray tube, and, if so, would it be full- or half-wave rectified if valve tubes I, II, and III burned out? II, III, and IV?

WORKSHEET 5-1 A BASIC X-RAY CIRCUIT

PURPOSE

Construct a basic x-ray circuit from basic electrical devices.

FOR FURTHER REVIEW

Refer to Chapter 5 in the accompanying textbook for further review of this topic.

ACTIVITIES

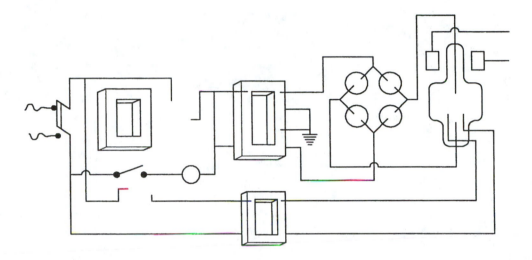

1. Draw in the appropriate coils for the three transformers to clearly indicate step-up, step-down, and autotransformers. Label each transformer's primary and secondary side as well as its type (i.e., step-up, etc.).

2. Draw in the mA control.

3. Draw in the diodes of the rectification circuit.

4. Draw in the anode and cathode of the x-ray tube.

5. Draw in a meter to measure the line voltage, amperage, and milliamperage.

6. Beginning at the main power breaker, draw arrows to indicate the flow of electrons through the complete circuit and draw a photon exiting the x-ray tube if your circuit would produce x-rays.

LABORATORY 5-2 GENERATORS

PURPOSE

Demonstrate the actual output waveform of an x-ray generator and explain the difference between different types of generators.

FOR FURTHER REVIEW

Refer to Chapter 5 in the accompanying textbook for further review of this topic.

MATERIALS

1. Energized radiographic unit, single, and/or three phase

2. X-ray output detector (some digital exposure timers and dosimeters are equipped with a BNC connector and can be used in this capacity)

3. Coaxial cable equipped with BNC connectors

4. Storage oscilloscope

Suggested Exposure Factors

100 mA, 0.5 sec, 80 kVp, 25″ source-to-detector distance

PROCEDURES

1. Connect one end of the cable to the BNC output of the output detector and the other end to the BNC input on the oscilloscope.

2. Place the detector on the radiographic table and center the x-ray tube to the detector. Turn on the oscilloscope and set the sensitivity level so that the oscilloscope is activated at the beginning of the x-ray waveform. The oscilloscope kilovoltage and time division controls should be set so that the output waveform covers the screen. Test exposures will have to be made to verify the appropriate oscilloscope settings. Refer to the oscilloscope operating manual or your instructor for help in obtaining the appropriate settings.

3. Expose the detector using the suggested exposure factors and view the output signal on the oscilloscope.

4. Draw the output waveform displayed.

5. Repeat the previous steps using 90 kVp and using 70 kVp.

6. Draw the output waveforms displayed for kVp settings.

7. Repeat this activity using a generator with a different waveform.

RESULTS

1. Label the drawing of the output waveforms, including the generator type, kVp, mA, and exposure time used.

LABORATORY 5-2 (Continued)

ANALYSIS

1. Does the output waveform appear to match the theoretical waveform of the generator type used? (See Chapter 5 of the textbook.) Explain your answer.

2. Compare the three output waveform drawings for a single generator type. Do they appear different? If so, how and why do they appear different? If not, should they have appeared different? How should they have appeared?

3. What diagnostic value does viewing output waveforms have in regard to generator condition?

4. Explain the output difference among a single-phase 2-pulse, a three-phase 6-pulse, and a three-phase 12-pulse generator.

5. Compare and contrast high-frequency and three-phase 12-pulse generators with respect to their output and design.

6. Explain the difference between a falling load and a constant potential generator.

WORKSHEET 6–1 X–RAY TUBES

PURPOSE

Describe the basic components and operation of a modern x-ray tube.

FOR FURTHER REVIEW

Refer to Chapters 5 and 6 in the accompanying textbook for further review of this topic.

MATERIALS

Various x-ray tubes

ACTIVITIES

1. Label the components of the x-ray tube in the following drawing.

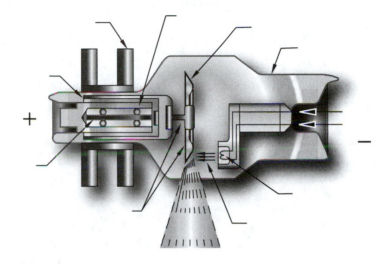

2. Examine the various x-ray tubes.

   a. Spin the anode and describe the sound (rough, smooth, etc.).

   b. Using a protractor, determine the angle of the anode(s) and record them.

   c. Identify the number of filaments in the cathode assembly for each tube.

   d. Describe any signs of tube wear or failure.

3. What is thermionic emission?

4. What is the function of the focusing cup?

5. What is the advantage of a rotating anode over a stationary anode?

6. Explain the line-focus principle.

7. How does the target angle affect the size of the effective focal spot? Draw a diagram to illustrate this concept.

8. Describe the anode heel effect.

9. How is the anode heel effect influenced by field size? distance?

WORKSHEET 6-2 RATING CHARTS AND COOLING CHARTS

PURPOSE

Determine safe tube exposures using a rating chart and a cooling chart.

FOR FURTHER REVIEW

Refer to Chapter 6 in the accompanying textbook for further review of this topic.

ACTIVITIES

1. Based on the following tube rating chart, circle the exposures that would be safe.

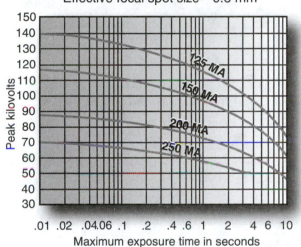

60 Hertz stator operation
Effective focal spot size—0.6 mm

Maximum exposure time in seconds

a. 125 mA, 0.4 sec, 120 kVp

b. 150 mA, 0.5 sec, 80 kVp

c. 150 mA, 2 sec, 100 kVp

d. 200 mA, 0.08 sec, 90 kVp

e. 200 mA, 0.1 sec, 70 kVp

f. 200 mA, 0.6 sec, 80 kVp

g. 250 mA, 0.2 sec, 70 kVp

h. 250 mA, 2 sec, 50 kVp

2. Based on the following tube rating chart below, circle the exposures that would be safe.

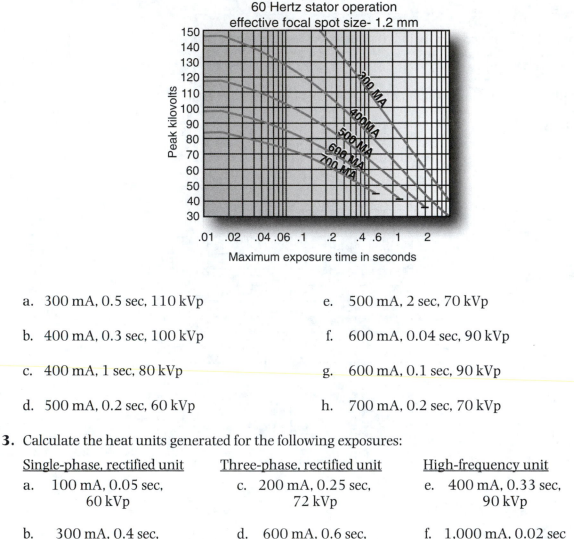

60 Hertz stator operation
effective focal spot size- 1.2 mm

Maximum exposure time in seconds

a. 300 mA, 0.5 sec, 110 kVp

b. 400 mA, 0.3 sec, 100 kVp

c. 400 mA, 1 sec, 80 kVp

d. 500 mA, 0.2 sec, 60 kVp

e. 500 mA, 2 sec, 70 kVp

f. 600 mA, 0.04 sec, 90 kVp

g. 600 mA, 0.1 sec, 90 kVp

h. 700 mA, 0.2 sec, 70 kVp

3. Calculate the heat units generated for the following exposures:

Single-phase, rectified unit	Three-phase, rectified unit	High-frequency unit
a. 100 mA, 0.05 sec, 60 kVp	c. 200 mA, 0.25 sec, 72 kVp	e. 400 mA, 0.33 sec, 90 kVp
b. 300 mA, 0.4 sec, 85 kVp	d. 600 mA, 0.6 sec, 88 kVp	f. 1,000 mA, 0.02 sec 120 kVp

WORKSHEET 6-2 (Continued)

Use the anode cooling chart that follows to answer the following questions.

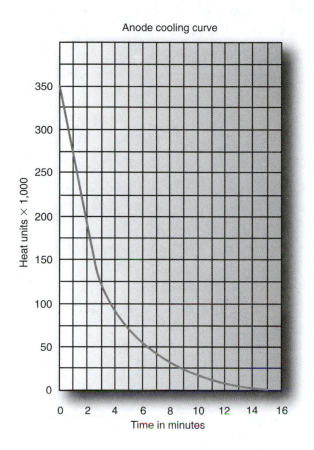

Anode cooling curve

4. Calculate the length of time necessary for the anode to cool to 25,000 heat units after 12 exposures of 600 mA, 0.2 sec at 70 kVp.

5. Calculate the length of time necessary for the anode to cool completely after 10 exposures of 1,000 mA, 0.05 sec at 80 kVp.

WORKSHEET 7–1 X-RAY PRODUCTION

PURPOSE

Explain the process of x-ray production.

FOR FURTHER REVIEW

Refer to Chapter 7 in the accompanying textbook for further review of this topic.

ACTIVITIES

1. What conditions are necessary for the production of x-rays?

2. What percentage of the kinetic energy of the electrons is converted to x-rays? What happens to the rest of the energy?

3. What are the two target interactions that can produce x-rays?

4. Study the following illustration

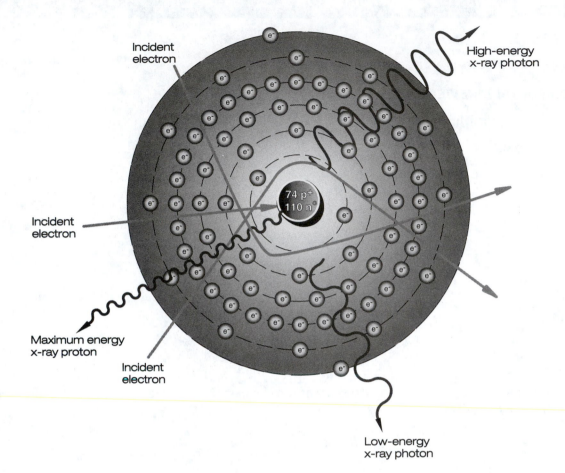

Incident electron

High-energy x-ray photon

74 p⁺ 110 n°

Incident electron

Maximum energy x-ray proton

Incident electron

Low-energy x-ray photon

a. What interaction is illustrated in the previous figure?

b. What determines the energy of the photon produced during this interaction?

WORKSHEET 7-1 (Continued)

5. Study the following illustration.

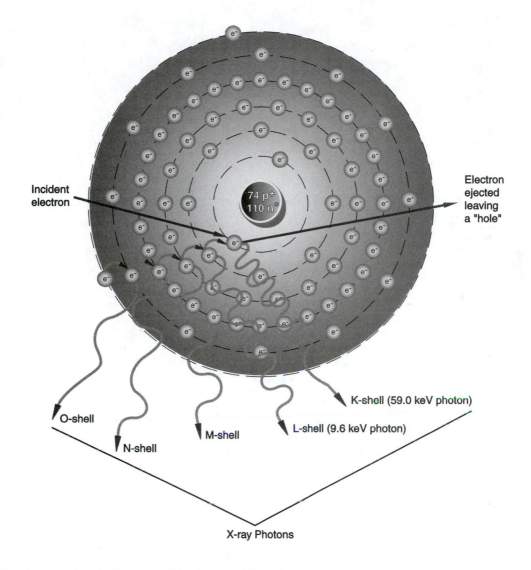

a. What interaction is illustrated in the preceding figure?

b. What determines the energy of the photon produced during this interaction?

6. What is meant by a characteristic cascade?

7. What is the K-shell binding energy for the following elements?

   a. molybdeum

   b. rhodium

   c. tungsten

8. What is meant by kilovoltage peak?

9. What is the relationship between the kilovoltage peak and the average energy (keV) of the photons in the primary beam?

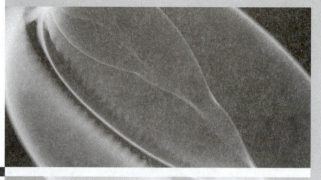

UNIT II   Protecting Patients
and Personnel

LABORATORY 8-1 USING DOSIMETRY EQUIPMENT

PURPOSE

Use basic ionizing radiation dosimetry equipment.

FOR FURTHER REVIEW

Refer to Chapter 8 in the accompanying textbook for further review of this topic.

MATERIALS

1. Energized radiographic unit

2. Abdomen phantom

3. Dosimeter

4. Ring stand

PROCEDURES

1. Position the abdomen phantom on the x-ray table. Use the ring stand to center the dosimeter directly over the sacrum at the point where the beam will enter the phantom.

2. Follow the instructions with the dosimetry equipment to record three exposures to the phantom.

RESULTS

1. Record the three exposures.

ANALYSIS

1. How close to one another were the three exposures?

2. What was the average exposure?

3. If exposures of 65 mR, 62 mR, and 131 mR were recorded, it would be advisable to perform three additional exposures. If the second set of exposures were 62 mR, 66 mR, and 65 mR, what would you record as the average exposure?

4. Why is it advised that the average of three exposures be used for all dosimetry measurements?

5. Why is the roentgen used as the unit of measurement?

WORKSHEET 8-2 UNITS AND MEASUREMENTS USED IN RADIATION PROTECTION

PURPOSE

Identify the types of ionizing radiation and the quantities and units used for the measurement of radiation.

FOR FURTHER REVIEW

Refer to Chapter 8 in the accompanying textbook for further review of this topic.

ACTIVITIES

Answer the following questions and solve the problems, showing your calculations.

Match the type of radiation to its description/characteristics.

a. x-ray   **b.** alpha   **c.** gamma   **d.** beta

———   **1.** can use a few cm of air as shield

———   **2.** electromagnetic radiation originating from a nucleus undergoing radioactive decay

———   **3.** is identical to a He nucleus

———   **4.** particulate radiation with a positive charge

———   **5.** electromagnetic radiation originating from the electron shells surrounding the nucleus

———   **6.** is identical to an electron

Match the appropriate unit to the statements below.

a. C/kg   **b.** sievert   **c.** kerma   **d.** gray   **e.** becquerel

———   **7.** equal to $Gy \times W_R$

———   **8.** unit of absorbed dose

———   **9.** applies only to x and γ radiation

———   **10.** unit of activity

———   **11.** equal to 1 joule/kg

———   **12.** exposure in air

———   **13.** takes into account the biological effectiveness of radiation

———   **14.** kinetic energy released per unit mass of matter

15. Using your own words, briefly explain the difference between absorbed dose and integral dose.

16. Using your own words, briefly explain the difference between equivalent dose and effective dose.

PROBLEMS

Convert the following units to their respective whole SI unit equivalents or to their respective whole conventional equivalents. Show calculations and include the appropriate units of measurement in your answer.

17. 145 mrem

18. 0.02 Sv

19. 10 cGy

20. 10 R

LABORATORY 9–1 BASIC RADIATION PROTECTION, DETECTION, AND MEASUREMENT

PURPOSE

Introduce commonly used radiation protection techniques and devices and demonstrate their effectiveness in reducing exposure to the patient and operator.

FOR FURTHER REVIEW

Refer to Chapter 9 in the accompanying textbook for further review of this topic.

MATERIALS

1. Energized radiographic unit (assumed to include about 2.5 mm/Al Eq filtration)

2. Abdomen phantom

3. Dosimeter

4. Flat contact gonad shields

5. Ring stand

PROCEDURES

1. Become familiar with the common radiation protection devices and techniques as introduced by your instructor.

2. Set up the x-ray tube and phantom as if to do an AP pelvis using a 40″ SID. Raise the phantom with sponges or sheets to create a tunnel large enough to accommodate the dosimeter ion chamber underneath the phantom.

    A. SOMATIC EXPOSURE—Entrance Skin Exposure (ESE)

    1. Effect of Filtration

        a. Center the ionization chamber on the anterior surface of the pelvis. Using a 14″ × 17″ field size, 70 kVp, and 60 mAs, expose and record ESE in mR on Table A.

        b. Center the ionization chamber on the posterior surface of the pelvis. Using a 14″ × 17″ field size, 70 kVp, and 60 mAs, expose and record the exit exposure in mR on Table A.

        c. Repeat 1a and 1b with 1 mm aluminum added to the primary beam for a total of about 3.5 mm Al.

        d. Repeat 1a and 1b with about 1 mm/Al filtration removed for a total of about 1.5 mm Al.

    2. Effect of kVp

        a. Repeat 1a and 1b but change the technique to 60 kVp and 120 mAs. (This new technique is a result of using the 15 percent rule in order to increase the contrast.)

        b. Repeat 1a and 1b but change the technique to 80 kVp and 30 mAs. (This new technique is a result of using the 15 percent rule in order to decrease the contrast.)

LABORATORY 9-1 (Continued)

B. GONAD EXPOSURE (MALE)

1. Use the ring stand to place the ionization chamber at the approximate location of the testes. Collimate the beam so the testes would be included in the beam. Using 70 kVp and 60 mAs, expose and record exposure in mR on table B.

2. Repeat B1 using a flat gonad shield placed over the area of the testes.

3. Repeat B1 with the beam collimated to the edge of the area of the testes. Do not use a shield.

4. Repeat B3 using a flat gonad shield placed over the area of the testes.

5. Repeat B1 using a collimated beam that excludes the area of the testes by 5 cm or more. Do not use the shield.

RESULTS

TABLE A

	kVp	mAs	SID	Total Filtration (Al Eq)	ESE (mR)	Exit Exposure (mR)
Effect of Filtration	70	60	40"	2.5 mm Al		
	70	60	40"	3.5 mm Al		
	70	60	40"	1.5 mm Al		
Effect of kVp	60	120	40"	2.5 mm Al		
	80	30	40"	2.5 mm Al		

TABLE B

	Exposure to Testes (mR)	
Beam Collimation	**No Shield**	**Shield**
Include Testes		
Exclude Testes		
Exclude Testes by 5 cm		XXXXXXXXXXXXXXXXX

LABORATORY 9-1 (Continued)

ANALYSIS

1. Which method(s) investigated reduced the ESEs to the pelvis?

2. Which method had the greatest effect on reducing the ESEs? Why do you think this method is so effective in reducing exposure?

3. Name two other possible methods that could be utilized in reducing the exposure to the patient.

4. List in order the protective methods used in the demonstration according to the gonad exposure received. List the most protective first. Briefly, why do you believe the list is arranged as it is?

5. Why is gonad shielding so important? Why are the male gonads more sensitive to exposure than the female gonads?

LABORATORY 10-1 EFFECTS OF FILTRATION

PURPOSE

Demonstrate the effect of filtration on x-ray emission.

FOR FURTHER REVIEW

Refer to Chapter 10 in the accompanying textbook for further review of this topic.

MATERIALS

1. Energized radiographic unit
2. Aluminum filters (0.25, 0.5, 1.0, 2.0 mm Al)
3. Dosimeter

SUGGESTED EXPOSURE FACTORS

100 mAs for three-phase generators and high-frequency generators, 60 kVp, 40″ SID

PROCEDURES

1. Center the dosimeter to the center of the x-ray field.

2. Direct the central ray perpendicular to the center of the dosimeter and collimate to a 4″ × 4″ field size.

3. Remove all added filtration from the x-ray tube. If this is not possible, the radiographic unit may be used as it is normally filtered. Expose the dosimeter.

4. Record the exposure received by the dosimeter as no aluminum added.

5. Add a 0.25 mm aluminum filter to the primary beam. The aluminum filters may be sequentially taped to the face of the collimator. Expose the dosimeter using the same exposure factors and record the exposure.

6. Add an additional 0.5 mm aluminum filter and repeat as listed in step 5. Follow the same procedures for 1.0 mm Al and 2.0 mm Al.

7. Reduce the mAs by 50% and repeat steps 1 through 8 using 90 kVp.

RESULTS

Dosimeter readings

Filtration	60 kVp	90 kVp
no aluminum added	____mR	____mR
0.25 mm aluminum	____mR	____mR
0.5 mm aluminum	____mR	____mR
1.0 mm aluminum	____mR	____mR
2.0 mm aluminum	____mR	____mR

LABORATORY 10-1 (Continued)

ANALYSIS

1. Based on the results obtained, what is the effect of adding filtration on x-ray emission? What would be the effect on radiographic density?

2. What is the purpose of filtering the radiographic beam?

3. What is the difference among inherent filtration, added filtration, and total filtration?

4. What is the most common filtering material used in diagnostic radiology?

5. What is the total filtration requirement for x-ray tubes that operate at above 70 kVp?

LABORATORY 10-2 HALF-VALUE LAYER DETERMINATION

PURPOSE

Calculate the half-value layer of a given x-ray unit.

FOR FURTHER REVIEW

Refer to Chapter 10 in the accompanying textbook for further review of this topic.

MATERIALS

1. Energized radiographic unit
2. 4 Aluminum attenuators (1.0 mm Al sheets)
3. Dosimeter

SUGGESTED EXPOSURE FACTORS

100 mAs for three-phase generators, 200 mAs for single-phase generators, 80 kVp, 40″ SID

PROCEDURES

1. Center the dosimeter ionization chamber to the center of the x-ray field. Collimate to a 4″ × 4″ field size.

2. Expose the dosimeter using the suggested exposure factors and record the exposure received by the dosimeter.

3. Form a shelf below the collimator by loosely taping a 1 mm Al attenuator to the collimator housing. This shelf will be used to hold additional Al attenuators. **NOTE: Make sure the Al attenuator intercepts the entire field of the collimator light. Repeat step 2.**

4. In sequence, add three 1.0 mm Al attenuators to the shelf, repeating step 2 after adding each one.

RESULTS

Dosimeter readings

Filtration	80 kVp
no aluminum added	_____mR
1 mm aluminum added	_____mR
2 mm aluminum added	_____mR
3 mm aluminum added	_____mR
4 mm aluminum added	_____mR

ANALYSIS

1. Plot calculated mR values versus total thickness of the Al attenuators added to the x-ray beam, on semilog graph paper. Draw a straight line through the plotted data points. The thickness of added Al attenuators that reduces the exposure output with 0 mm Al added by one-half is the measured half-value layer. What is the measured half-value layer?

2. A single-phase x-ray tube with a total filtration of 2.5 mm Al/Eq should produce an x-ray beam with a half-value layer of 2.4 mm Al using 80 kVp. A three-phase x-ray tube with a total filtration of 2.5 mm Al/Eq should produce an x-ray beam with a half-value layer of 2.7 mm Al using 80 kVp. Explain why the recommended half-value layers are different.

3. What are some of the possible causes for the HVL being less than that recommended? What is/are the practical implication(s) of this situation?

4. What are some of the possible causes for the HVL being excessively large in comparison to the recommended value? What is/are the practical implication(s) of this situation?

5. Define *half-value layer.*

WORKSHEET 11-1 CALCULATING PRIME FACTORS

PURPOSE

Perform calculations to adjust the various prime factors.

FOR FURTHER REVIEW

Refer to Chapter 11 in the accompanying textbook for further review of this topic.

ACTIVITIES

1. Given the following mA and exposure times, calculate the mAs.

	mA	time		mAs
a.	200	1/40	=	_____
b.	400	3/10	=	_____
c.	300	3/5	=	_____
d.	100	1/20	=	_____
e.	600	1/4	=	_____
f.	100	0.05	=	_____
g.	400	0.017	=	_____
h.	300	0.20	=	_____
i.	200	0.33	=	_____
j.	1,000	0.006	=	_____

2. Given the following mAs and mA values, calculate the exposure time.

	mA	time		mAs
a.	100	_____	=	75
b.	300	_____	=	120
c.	200	_____	=	5
d.	600	_____	=	15
e.	400	_____	=	80

3. Given the following mAs and exposure time values, calculate the mA.

	mA	time		mAs
a.	____	0.03	=	30
b.	____	0.05	=	35
c.	____	0.7	=	210
d.	____	1/4	=	75
e.	____	1/10	=	60

4. Using the inverse square law, calculate the new exposure when the distance is changed.

a. 36-inch SID   40-inch SID
    250 mR   ____mR

b. 28-inch SID   42-inch SID
    175 mR   ____mR

c. 36-inch SID   72-inch SID
    100 mR   ____mR

d. 40-inch SID   72-inch SID
    125 mR   ____mR

e. 40-inch SID   56-inch SID
    80 mR   ____mR

5. Using the exposure (film density) maintenance formula, calculate the missing factor.

a. 40-inch SID   72-inch SID
    40 mAs   ____mAs

b. 72-inch SID   36-inch SID
    75 mAs   ____mAs

c. 40-inch SID   56-inch SID
    160 mAs   ____mAs

d. 40-inch SID   ____SID
    12 mAs   27 mAs

e. 72-inch SID   ____SID
    20 mAs   10 mAs

6. Using the 15 percent image receptor exposure/rule, calculate the kVp that will produce the same image receptor exposure as the original set of factors.

a. 150 mAs   300 mAs
    60 kVp   ____kVp

b. 25 mAs   50 mAs
    80 kVp   ____kVp

c. 60 mAs   120 mAs
    75 kVp   ____kVp

d. 200 mAs   100 mAs
    90 kVp   ____kVp

e. 10 mAs   5 mAs
    50 kVp   ____kVp

LABORATORY 11-2 EFFECT OF mAs, kVp, AND SID ON X-RAY EMISSION

PURPOSE

Demonstrate the effect of mAs, kVp, and SID on x-ray emission.

FOR FURTHER REVIEW

Refer to Chapter 11 in the accompanying textbook for further review of this topic.

MATERIALS

1. Energized radiographic unit

2. Dosimeter

SUGGESTED EXPOSURE FACTORS

100 mA, 0.1 sec, 10 mAs, 50 kVp, 36″ SID

PROCEDURES

1. Place the dosimeter ion chamber in the center of the x-ray beam.

2. Direct the central ray perpendicular to the center of the ion chamber and collimate to a 5″ × 5″ field size.

3. Expose the ion chamber and record the results.

mAs/X-Ray Emission

4. Repeat steps 1 through 3, changing the suggested factors to 20 mAs.

5. Repeat steps 1 through 3, changing the suggested factors to 30 mAs.

kVp/X-Ray Emission

6. Repeat steps 1 through 3, changing the suggested factors to 60 kVp.

7. Repeat steps 1 through 3, changing the suggested factors to 70 kVp.

SID/X-Ray Emission

8. Repeat steps 1 through 3, changing the suggested factors to 56″ SID.

9. Repeat steps 1 through 3, changing the suggested exposure factors to 72″ SID.

RESULTS

1. Record the dosimeter readings:

   Initial exposure _____

   mAs/X-RAY EMISSION

        20 mAs _____   30 mAs _____

   kVp/X-RAY EMISSION

        60 kVp _____   70 kVp _____

   SID/X-RAY EMISSION

        56″ SID _____   72″ SID _____

ANALYSIS

mAs/X-Ray Emission

1. What effect does increasing mAs have on the exposure?

2. What is the specific relationship between mAs and x-ray emission?

kVp/X-Ray Emission

3. What effect does increasing kVp have on exposure?

4. What is the specific relationship between kVp and x-ray emission?

SID/X-Ray Emission

5. What effect does increasing SID have on x-ray exposure?

6. What is the specific relationship between SID and x-ray emission?

WORKSHEET 12–1 X–RAY INTERACTIONS

PURPOSE

Explain the interactions between x-rays and matter.

FOR FURTHER REVIEW

Refer to Chapter 12 in the accompanying textbook for further review of this topic.

ACTIVITIES

1. Draw a diagram to illustrate the photoelectric interaction between x-ray and matter.

2. How is secondary radiation produced?

3. Draw a diagram to illustrate the Compton interaction between x-ray and matter.

4. How is scatter radiation produced?

5. What is the predominant interaction in the diagnostic x-ray range?

6. What is the relationship of kVp to the incidence of x-ray interaction?

7. How does kVp affect the number of photoelectric versus Compton interactions?

8. How does scatter radiation affect image contrast?

9. Explain the process of coherent scattering.

10. Discuss the role of coherent scattering in diagnostic imaging.

LABORATORY 13-1 ESTIMATING PATIENT ENTRANCE SKIN EXPOSURE

PURPOSE

Estimate entrance skin exposure (ESE) for various radiographic projections.

FOR FURTHER READING

Refer to Chapter 13 in the accompanying textbook for further review of this topic.

MATERIALS

1. Energized radiographic unit
2. Digital dosimeter
3. Technique chart

PROCEDURES

1. Obtain a reliable technique chart (ideally one that is used in clinical practice) and, using the techniques from the chart, calculate the ESE values for a 23 cm PA chest, 15 cm lateral skull, 23 cm AP abdomen, 23 cm AP L-Spine, and a 13 cm AP C-Spine according to the following steps.

2. Set the tube SID at the appropriate distance for the projection, place the dosimeter's ion chamber detector on the radiographic table, center, and collimate the beam to the appropriate part size. Set the exposure factors according to the chart, turn on the digital dosimeter unit, select the single-dose mode, and follow the manufacturer's instructions, record an exposure.

3. Determine the thickness of the detector and the distance from the Bucky tray to the table top (part image receptor distance) in cm. Use these figures to determine the source-to-skin distance (SSD) and the source-to-detector distance (SDD).

4. Use the inverse square law to determine the ESE delivered to the body part.

$$\frac{\text{Dosimeter exposure reading (mR)}}{\text{ESE (mR)}} = \frac{\text{SSD}^2}{\text{SDD}^2}$$

Grid Techniques

SSD = SID − (part thickness + part image receptor distance)

SDD = SID − (detector thickness + part image receptor distance)

Table Top Techniques

SSD = SID − part thickness

SDD = SID − detector thickness

LABORATORY 13-1 (Continued)

RESULTS

1. Record your data below.

	Dosimeter Exposure (mR)	SSD (cm)	SDD (cm)	ESE (mR)
AP chest	____	____	____	____
Lateral skull	____	____	____	____
AP abdomen	____	____	____	____
AP C-Spine	____	____	____	____
AP L-Spine	____	____	____	____

ANALYSIS

1. What is the ESE for the five projections?

2. Compare your ESE results with the Conference of Radiation Control Program Directors Average Patient Exposure Guides in the textbook.

3. Describe three ways that ESE can be reduced.

4. What correlations can be drawn about ESE and organ dose?

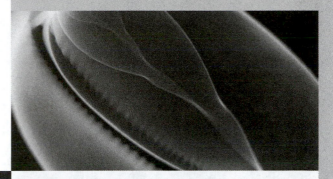

UNIT III Creating the Image

LABORATORY 14-1 THINKING THREE-DIMENSIONALLY

PURPOSE

Illustrate the importance of multiple projections in perceiving the radiographic image as representation of a three-dimensional object.

FOR FURTHER REVIEW

Refer to Chapter 14 in the accompanying textbook for further review of this topic.

MATERIALS

1. Energized radiographic unit

2. Chest phantom with hollow lung fields is preferred although a solid chest, abdomen, or pelvis phantom can be substituted

3. 14″ × 17″ cassette with image receptor

4. Dosimeter

5. Film processor

SUGGESTED EXPOSURE FACTORS

Chest: 400 RS, 4 mAs, 80 kVp, 72″ SID, nongrid
Abdomen: 400 RS, 20 mAs, 80 kVp, 40″ SID, 8:1 Bucky grid

PROCEDURES

1. The instructor prepares the phantom by taping several artifacts (keys, hairpins, paper clips, etc.) onto the phantom, at least one each on the surface located anterior, posterior, right lateral, left lateral, and opposite obliques (i.e., right posterior and left anterior surfaces). When a hollow chest phantom can be used, half the artifacts should be inside the chest wall and half outside. Each artifact must be located at a separate superior-inferior location so that no two artifacts will be superimposed on AP, oblique, or lateral radiographs. The prepared phantom is then covered with a patient gown to hide artifact locations from students.

2. Chest phantom: Place the phantom vertically on the tabletop and center it to a loaded cassette held vertical in a cassette holder.

   Abdomen/pelvis phantom: Place the phantom recumbent on the table and center it to a loaded cassette in the Bucky tray.

3. Direct the central ray perpendicular to the center of the film, position the phantom for an AP position, and collimate to the part.

4. Expose and process the film. Label the film by position.

5. Repeat steps 2 through 4 for a left lateral, LPO, and RPO position.

LABORATORY 14-1 (Continued)

RESULTS

1. Use a marker to number each artifact on all four films (i.e., label the first artifact #1 on the AP, lateral, and both oblique films, the second artifact #2 on each film, etc.).

ANALYSIS

1. Give the precise location of each artifact on the phantom. For example, specify location as to anterior, posterior, right or left lateral, RPO, LPO, LAO, RAO surface. For a hollow chest phantom, specify whether the artifact is located inside or outside the chest wall.

2. Give the minimum number of projections that are necessary to locate each artifact and explain why fewer projections would not define each location.

LABORATORY 15-1 BEAM RESTRICTION

PURPOSE

Demonstrate the effects of beam restriction on radiographic image quality.

FOR FURTHER REVIEW

Refer to Chapter 15 in the accompanying textbook for further review of this topic.

MATERIALS

1. Energized radiographic unit

2. Phantom knee

3. 2 water-filled plastic gallon jugs

4. $10'' \times 12''$ film/screen cassette

5. Automatic film processor

6. $10'' \times 12''$ CR cassette or DR

SUGGESTED EXPOSURE FACTORS

400 RS, 100 mA, 0.05 sec, 70 kVp, 40 SID, nongrid

PROCEDURES

1. Make two exposures of the knee in a PA position using a table top procedure and two $10'' \times 12''$ cassettes. Two water-filled jugs will be used to simulate extra tissue.

2. Center the cassette lengthwise to the table top. Center the knee to the cassette and place the water jugs on both sides. Center to the knee and open collimators to include as much of the water jugs as possible and expose.

3. Repeat step 2, but collimate the beam closely to include just the knee.

4. Process films.

5. Repeat step 2 using a CR cassette tabletop or a DR receptor, nongrid

6. Repeat step 5, but collimate the beam closely to include just the knee.

7. Process digital images.

RESULTS

1. Review the radiographs with respect to radiographic density and contrast differences exhibited.

LABORATORY 15-1 (Continued)

ANALYSIS

1. Which radiograph demonstrates the best image quality? Why?

2. Compare the quality of the four images

   a. What factor(s) cause a change in the quality between the two film/screen receptor images?

   b. What factor(s) cause a change in the quality between the two CR or DR receptor images?

   c. What factor(s) cause a change in the quality between the film/screen receptor and CR/DR images without collimation?

   d. What factor(s) cause a change in the quality between the film/screen receptor and CR/DR images with collimation?

   e. Which image displays the best quality? Why?

3. What patient-related factors contribute to the production of scatter radiation?

4. What x-ray beam related factors contribute to the production of scatter radiation?

5. Describe two different devices that are used in diagnostic radiology for beam restriction.

LABORATORY 16-1 EFFECT OF SUBJECT ON ATTENUATION AND SCATTER

PURPOSE

Demonstrate the effect of subject thickness on attenuation and scatter of the primary x-ray beam.

FOR FURTHER REVIEW

Refer to Chapter 16 in the accompanying textbook for further review of this topic.

MATERIALS

1. Energized radiographic unit

2. Automatic film processor

3. Abdomen phantom

4. 14″ × 17″ radiographic cassettes with image receptor

5. 14″ × 17″ wire mesh test tool

6. Cassette holder

7. Dosimeter

SUGGESTED EXPOSURE FACTORS

20 mAs, 95 kVp, 40″ SID, nongrid

PROCEDURES

1. Place the abdomen phantom in an AP position on sponges or sheets high enough to create a tunnel of sufficient height to permit the placement of the dosimeter chamber underneath the phantom. Center the phantom to the table top with the central ray perpendicular to the level of the iliac crest and collimate to the abdomen. Place the dosimeter detector on the anterior surface of the abdomen at the location of the central ray and expose. Record the dosimeter reading in mR as the entrance exposure.

2. Repeat step 1, but place the dosimeter detector at the posterior surface of the phantom at the location of the central ray. Record the dosimeter reading in mR as the exit exposure.

3. Place the wire mesh test tool on top of a loaded 14″ × 17″ cassette. Secure both crosswise in a vertical position using a cassette holder as shown in the following figure. Position the cassette holder so that the cassette is approximately 1 inch from the lateral edge of the phantom and centered to the level of the iliac crest. Using a perpendicular central ray, center the tube to the level of the iliac crest and collimate the beam to the abdomen. The primary beam should not include any portion of the vertical cassette. Expose the phantom using the technique in step 1 and process the image receptor.

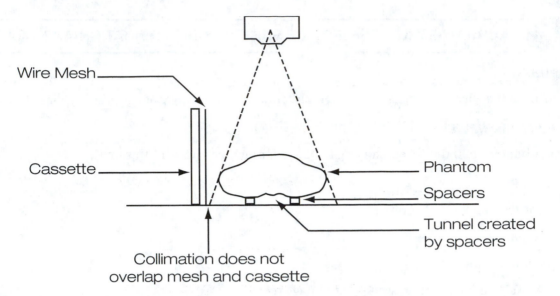

4. Position the phantom for a lateral abdomen. Center a perpendicular central ray to the level of the iliac crest and collimate to the phantom, using a 40″ SID. Place the dosimeter detector on the superior lateral surface of the phantom at the location of the central ray. Expose using 5 mAs at 95 kVp. Record the dosimeter reading in mR as the entrance exposure.

5. Repeat step 4, but place the dosimeter detector at the inferior lateral surface of the phantom at the location of the central ray. Record the dosimeter reading in mR as the exit exposure.

6. Place the wire mesh test tool on top of a loaded 14″ × 17″ cassette. Secure both crosswise in a vertical position using a cassette holder. Position the cassette holder so that the cassette is approximately 1 inch from the posterior surface of the phantom and centered to the level of the iliac crest. Using a perpendicular central ray, center it to the level of the iliac crest and collimate the beam to the phantom. The primary beam should not include the vertical cassette. Expose the phantom using the technique in step 4 and process the film.

7. Use a densitometer to measure the optical density at the center of the bottom, middle, and top thirds of both radiographs. Record the readings.

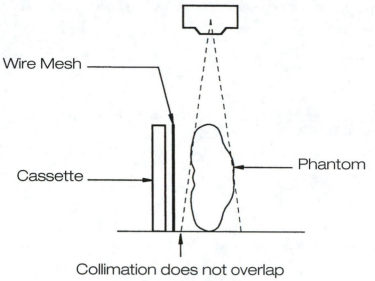

Wire Mesh

Cassette

Phantom

Collimation does not overlap
mesh and cassette

RESULTS

Attenuation

Projection	Part Thickness	Entrance Exposure (mR)	Exit Exposure (mR)
AP Abdomen	_____	_____	_____
Lat Abdomen	_____	_____	_____

Scatter

| Projection | Part Thickness | OD Image Receptor | | |
		Bottom Third	Middle Third	Top Third
AP Abdomen	_____	_____	_____	_____
Lat Abdomen	_____	_____	_____	_____

ANALYSIS

1. Were the entrance exposures similar or different for the AP and lateral abdomen? Why?

LABORATORY 16-1 (Continued)

2. Were the exit exposures similar or different for the AP and lateral abdomen? Why?

3. Which radiograph showed the greatest amount of radiographic image receptor exposure? Why?

4. Were you able to demonstrate a difference between the radiographic image receptor exposures produced on the bottom, middle, and top thirds of the AP abdomen radiograph? If so, how would you explain this?

5. Were you able to demonstrate a difference between the radiographic image receptor exposures produced on the bottom, middle, and top thirds of the lateral abdomen radiograph? If so, how would you explain this?

6. What happens to the quality and quantity of the beam as it passes from entrance to exit through the patient? How were these effects demonstrated on the radiographs you produced as part of this lab?

7. List all the subject-related factors that would have a bearing on attenuation and scatter of the beam.

8. Are there factors besides the subject that affect the attenuation and scatter of the beam? Explain.

LABORATORY 17-1 THE EFFECT OF PATHOLOGY ON IMAGE QUALITY

PURPOSE

Illustrate the effect of pathology on image quality.

FOR FURTHER REVIEW

Refer to Chapter 17 in the accompanying textbook for further review of this topic.

MATERIALS

Radiographs demonstrating:

Chest
Congestive heart failure
Emphysema
Pleural effusion
Pneumonia
Pneumothorax
Tuberculosis

Abdomen
Ascites
Bowel obstruction

Extremities/Skull
Active osteomyelitis
Degenerative arthritis
Osteoporosis
Paget's disease

ACTIVITIES

1. Based on a review of the radiographs, which of the images demonstrates an increased attenuation (additive) condition?

2. What causes a pathologic condition to result in an increased attenuation of the x-ray beam?

3. Based on a review of the radiographs, which of the images demonstrates a decreased attenuation (destructive) condition?

4. What causes a pathologic condition to result in a decreased attenuation of the x-ray beam?

5. Based on a review of the radiographs, which images required an adjustment from normal technical factors used for the procedure?

6. What technical factor adjustments are recommended for additive conditions? For destructive conditions?

LABORATORY 18-1 GRID COMPARISONS AND CONVERSIONS

PURPOSE

Demonstrate the use of grid conversion factors.

FOR FURTHER REVIEW

Refer to Chapter 18 in the accompanying textbook for further review of this topic.

MATERIALS

1. Energized radiographic unit

2. Automatic film processor

3. 8:1 and 12:1 radiographic grids

4. Abdomen phantom

5. Cassettes with image receptor

6. Step wedge (penetrometer)

7. Densitometer

SUGGESTED EXPOSURE FACTORS

400 RS, 200 mA, 0.03 sec, 75 kVp, 40″ SID, nongrid

PROCEDURES

1. Center the abdomen phantom to the image receptor on the tabletop. Place the step wedge beside the phantom on the image receptor. Direct the central ray perpendicular to the center of the image receptor and collimate to the edges.

2. Use the suggested factors to expose the image receptor, process, and label it #1. Use a densitometer to measure the OD of step 5. If it is not 1.2 ± 0.2, adjust the mAs and reexpose.

3. Repeat step 1 using an 8:1 ratio grid. Expose the image receptor using the appropriate grid conversion factor, process, and label it #2. If it is not 1.2 ± 0.2, adjust the mAs and reexpose.

4. Repeat step 1 using a 12:1 ratio grid. Expose the image receptor using the appropriate grid conversion factor, process, and label it #3. If it is not 1.2 ± 0.2, adjust the mAs and reexpose.

5. Use a densitometer to measure the OD (optical density) of step 5 on the step wedge for all the images and record the readings in the results section.

LABORATORY 18–1 (Continued)

RESULTS

1. Review the three images in terms of their exposure.

<u>Step 5 Optical Density (OD)</u>

Image #1   _____

Image #2   _____

Image #3   _____

ANALYSIS

1. When is it necessary to use a radiographic grid for an examination?

2. Describe the appearance of images 1, 2, and 3. Which one(s) more closely approximate(s) a quality image? Why?

3. Where were the exposures of the three images the same? If they were not, were the differences significant? Explain.

4. Based on your data, what conclusions can you draw about the effect of grids and grid ratios on conversion factors?

5. What factors or influences contribute to the decrease or increase of image quality in each of the images?

6. Based on the procedure, what is the importance of a radiographic grid?

Name _____ Course _____ Date _____

LABORATORY 18-2 GRID ERRORS

PURPOSE

Demonstrate the effects of the common errors accompanying the use of radiographic grids.

FOR FURTHER REVIEW

Refer to Chapter 18 in the accompanying textbook for further review of this topic.

MATERIALS

1. Energized radiographic unit
2. Automatic film processor
3. 12:1 80 line/inch linear focused grid
4. Cassettes with image receptor
5. Skull phantom

SUGGESTED EXPOSURE FACTORS

400 RS, 50 mA, 0.15 sec, 80 kVp, 40″ SID, 12:1 stationary grid

PROCEDURES

1. Center a 10″ × 12″ stationary linear focused grid on a 10″ × 12″ loaded cassette placed crosswise in the center of a radiographic table. Position the phantom skull for a lateral projection, making sure the perpendicular CR is directed to the center of the grid. Expose using the suggested exposure factors.

2. Process the image receptor and label it exposure #1.

3. Repeat step 1, but move the perpendicular CR approximately 3″ toward the top of the skull so that it is off center of the grid center line. Open the collimator sufficiently to expose the entire cassette. Process the image receptor and label it exposure #2.

4. Repeat step 1, but angle the CR caudally 15° across the grid's center line with it centered to the grid. Adjust the SID to compensate for the angulation and open the collimator sufficiently to expose the entire cassette. Process the image receptor and label it exposure #3.

5. Repeat step 1, but elevate the side of the cassette under the chin 15° from the plane of the table using a positioning sponge. Adjust the phantom skull to maintain its lateral position. Process the image receptor and label it exposure #4.

6. Repeat step 1, but turn the grid upside down. Make sure the CR is centered to the grid. Process the image receptor and label it exposure #5.

7. Repeat step 1, but use a 50″ SID. Process the image receptor and label it exposure #6.

8. Repeat step 1, but use a 30″ SID. Process the image receptor and label it exposure #7.

LABORATORY 18-2 (Continued)

RESULTS

1. Using image #1 as the standard for comparison, review the six images with respect to image quality.

ANALYSIS

1. Describe images 2 through 7 with respect to their image quality.

2. Which grid error(s) had the worst effect on the image quality? Explain the reason for this occurrance.

3. Which grid error(s) had the least effect on the image quality? Explain the reason for this occurrance.

4. Would you expect the results to be more or less severe with a lower ratio grid? Justify your answer.

5. Based on the results of the experiment, state at least four rules that should be followed when using linear focused grids.

LABORATORY 18-3 THE AIR GAP TECHNIQUE

PURPOSE

Demonstrate the effects of the air gap technique on radiographic image quality.

FOR FURTHER REVIEW

Refer to Chapter 18 in the accompanying textbook for further review of this topic.

MATERIALS

1. Energized radiographic unit

2. Automatic film processor

3. Skull phantom

4. 10″ × 12″ cassettes with image receptor

5. Densitometer

SUGGESTED EXPOSURE FACTORS

400 RS, 100 mA, .04 sec, 80 kVp, 40″ SID, nongrid

PROCEDURES

1. Position the skull phantom for a lateral projection using a 10″ × 12″ cassette crosswise on the tabletop. Center and collimate the beam to the cassette. Expose the image receptor using the suggested exposure factors, process, and label it #1.

2. Repeat step 1 with the skull elevated 7″ above the cassette. Use positioning sponges or other appropriate means to achieve this effect. Expose, process the image, and label it #2.

3. Measure and record the optical density of the sella turcica for each image using a densitometer.

RESULTS

1. Visually review and compare the two images with regard to their image quality.

2. Record the optical density measurements of the sella turcica.

                              Optical Density (OD)

    Skull in contact with cassette (#1)   _____
    Skull with 7″ air gap (#2)   _____

LABORATORY 18-3 (Continued)

ANALYSIS

1. Was there a difference in the optical densities of the sella turcica on the two images? If so, was the difference significant? Explain the reason for the difference.

2. Describe any other differences between the images that are apparent and explain the reason(s) for the difference(s).

3. When an air gap is present, what can a radiographer do in order to reduce loss of image sharpness?

4. Give at least two clinical applications for the air gap technique and explain the rationale for its use in each case.

LABORATORY 18-4 THE MOIRE EFFECT WHEN UTILIZING COMPUTED RADIOGRAPHIC SYSTEMS

PURPOSE

To demonstrate the appearance and cause of a moire effect grid artifact when utilizing CR imaging systems.

FOR FURTHER REVIEW

Refer to Chapter 18 in the accompanying textbook for further review of this topic.

MATERIALS

1. Energized radiographic unit

2. 2 - 10″ × 12″ CR cassette

3. Skull phantom

4. 8:1 ratio 10″ × 12″ stationary linear (LD) grid with a frequency higher than 178 lines/inch

5. 8:1 ratio 10″ × 12″ stationary linear (LD) grid with a frequency lower than 178 lines/inch

SUGGESTED EXPOSURE FACTORS

80 kVp, 10 mAs, 40″ SID

PROCEDURES

1. Position the skull for a lateral skull using a 10″ × 12″ cassette and the 8:1 ration grid with a frequency higher than 178 lines/inch crosswise (landscape) on the tabletop. Center and collimate the beam to the cassette. Exposure the cassette and process it using a lateral skull algorithm, marking the image "#1>178 crosswise."

2. Repeat step 1 using the 8:1 ratio grid with a frequency lower than 178 lines/inch. Expose the cassette and process it using a lateral skull algorithm, marking the image "#2<178 crosswise."

3. Repeat step 1, placing the cassette and grid in a vertical (portrait) position. Expose the cassette and process it using a lateral skull algorithm, marking the image "#3>178 vertical."

4. Repeat step 2, placing the cassette and grid in a vertical (portrait) position, Expose the cassette and process it using a lateral skull algorithm, marking the image "#4<178 vertical."

RESULTS

1. Visually review and compare the four skull images with regard to image quality.

2. Record the exposure index for each image.

ANALYSIS

1. Was there a difference in the appearance of grid lines on the four images? If so, is the difference significant?

2. Which grid had the worst effect on image quality? Explain the reason for this occurrence.

3. Does placing the grid in a vertical (portrait) vs. crosswise (landscape) change the appearance of the image in terms of grid artifact? Why or why not?

WORKSHEET 19-1 RADIOGRAPHIC FILM

PURPOSE

Describe the construction of radiographic film, the formation of the latent image, and the different types of radiographic film.

FOR FURTHER REVIEW

Refer to Chapter 19 in the accompanying textbook for further review of this topic.

ACTIVITIES

Answer the following questions.

Film Construction

1. Draw a cross section of a radiographic film and label all the layers.

2. The film base that provides the increased strength and thinner form needed for automatic processing is:

   a. cellulose nitrate   c. polyester

   b. cellulose acetate   d. glass

3. The emulsion of a radiographic film is composed of silver halide and:

   a. cellulose   c. gelatin

   b. polyester   d. an adhesive

4. Composition of radiographic film. Mark each item True (T) or False (F).

   _____ a. Modern radiographic film has a polyester base.

   _____ b. A faint blue dye is added to the film base to enhance radiographic contrast.

   _____ c. Medical radiographic film has a double emulsion.

   _____ d. Gelatin is used in the emulsion because it has the ability to swell and absorb the processing chemicals without dissolving.

   _____ e. The protective coating helps to prevent artifacts that may result from film handling.

5. Film speed is mainly determined by the _____ of silver halide crystals, and the _____ of the emulsion layer.

6. Silver bromide is formed as a result of the combination of silver nitrate and _____.

7. The atoms comprising the silver halide crystal are bound together by _____ bonds.

Latent Image

Mark each item True (T) or False (F).

_____ **1.** The latent image is a speck of silver on a silver bromide crystal capable of initiating development of the entire crystal.

_____ **2.** The latent image is formed when positively charged interstitial silver ions combine with trapped electrons at the sensitivity speck.

_____ **3.** The sensitivity speck is composed of silver sulfide.

_____ **4.** After exposure to radiant energy, the film emulsion is more susceptible to handling artifacts.

_____ **5.** Theoretically, three or more atoms of silver must be deposited at the sensitivity speck to form a stable latent image.

Film Types

Match the film types in column A with the correct characteristics listed in column B.

Column A—Film Type   Column B—Characteristics

_____ **1.** Nonscreen / Direct exposure

_____ **2.** Mammography

_____ **3.** Screen

_____ **4.** Orthochromatic

_____ **5.** Fluoroscopic photospot

_____ **6.** Duplicating

_____ **7.** Video imaging

_____ **8.** Laser

_____ **9.** Panchromatic

a. Most sensitive to the spectral emission of radiographic intensifying screens

b. Sensitive to the blue through green portion of visible light spectrum

c. Sensitive to the light emitted by a CRT

d. Fine grain infrared sensitive

e. Sensitive to the entire visible light spectrum

f. Small format (70 to 105 mm) roll or cut film that can be processed and viewed like conventional radiographs

g. Fine grain single emulsion film used with single screened cassettes

h. Relatively thick single emulsion layer, which is used for special applications

i. Solarized film that is sensitive to ultraviolet light

WORKSHEET 19-2 LATENT IMAGE FORMATION

PURPOSE

Describe latent image formation.

FOR FURTHER REVIEW

Refer to Chapter 19 in the accompanying textbook for further review of this topic.

ACTIVITIES

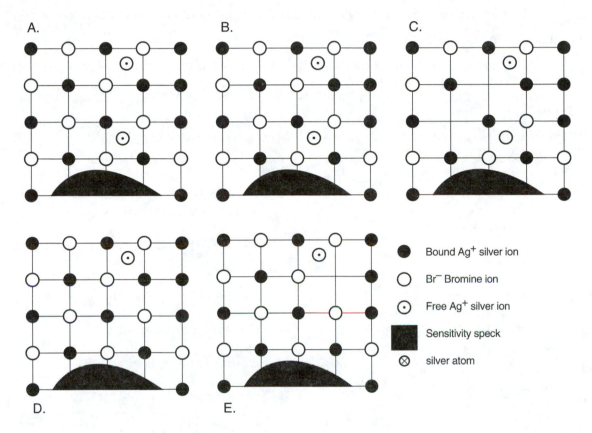

1. On Figure A draw an incident photon striking a bromide ion. Also draw an electron ejected from the resulting interaction.

2. On Figure B draw the ejected electron where it migrates after the interaction.

3. On Figure C draw the movement of a free silver ion to the sensitivity speck.

4. On Figure D show the final step in the process of latent image formation.

5. On Figure E show an accumulation large enough to result in a black metallic silver deposit when development occurs.

6. What type of interaction must occur between the incident photon and the bromide ion in Figure A?

7. Where does the ejected electron migrate in Figure B?

8. Why is the free silver ion attracted to the sensitivity speck in Figure C?

9. What occurs in Figure D?

WORKSHEET 19-3 RADIOGRAPHIC FILM HANDLING AND STORAGE

PURPOSE

Describe the handling and storage of radiographic film.

FOR FURTHER REVIEW

Refer to Chapter 19 in the accompanying textbook for further review of this topic.

ACTIVITIES

Answer the following questions.

1. Boxed radiographic film should be stored _____ in order to prevent pressure artifacts on the film.

2. Opened boxes of film should be stored at _____°F or less and between _____ percent and _____ percent relative humidity.

3. Define film artifact.

4. List four different causes of film artifacts.

5. What is base plus fog? List three environmental conditions that may affect base plus fog levels.

6. Why must darkrooms have stricter shielding requirements than exposure rooms?

7. Explain what is meant by "rotating film stock"? Why is it necessary to do so?

LABORATORY 19-4 CASSETTE AND FILM HANDLING

PURPOSE

Demonstrate artifacts that result from common film mishandling situations.

FOR FURTHER REVIEW

Refer to Chapter 19 in the accompanying textbook for further review of this topic.

MATERIALS

1. Automatic film processor
2. Hand lotion
3. Radiographic film

PROCEDURES

1. Under darkroom conditions, lay a single sheet of fresh film on the darkroom bench. Pick up the film and grasp it between your thumb and the first two fingers of one hand. Make a conscious effort to squeeze and kink the film. Next drop the film on the darkroom floor, slide it across the floor, and step on it.

2. Apply some hand lotion to your fingers. Pick up the film and grasp one edge with your fingers. Wipe the lotion off your fingers and wet your hands. Pick up the film and grasp the other edge with your wet fingers, then process the film.

RESULTS

1. Review the processed film for the presence of artifacts.

ANALYSIS

1. What is a film artifact? Why are they of concern?

2. Describe the artifacts present on the film. Match each artifact with the mishandling that caused it.

3. Describe other artifacts that can occur due to rough handling.

LABORATORY 19-5 RADIOGRAPHIC DUPLICATION AND LIGHTENING TECHNIQUES

PURPOSE

Duplicate a diagnostic quality image accurately and correct an image that is too dark by overexposing duplication film.

FOR FURTHER REVIEW

Refer to Chapter 19 in the accompanying textbook for further review of this topic.

MATERIALS

1. Diagnostic quality image

2. Image that is approximately 2 to 3× too dark

3. Radiographic duplication unit

4. Duplication film

5. Automatic film processor

6. Densitometer

EXPOSURE FACTORS

Suggested Factors
1 to 2 seconds

PROCEDURES

Duplication

1. Use the procedure detailed in Figure 19-7 in the textbook to duplicate the diagnostic quality image.

Lightening

1. Use 15 seconds more than the exposure time that produced the duplicate film to duplicate the dark image.

2. Continue to duplicate the dark image at 15-second exposure increases until a diagnostic quality duplicate has been produced.

RESULTS

Duplication

1. Select an average density area on the diagnostic quality image (i.e., soft tissue between the sacrum and body of L5 on an abdomen, lung field between 3rd and 4th ribs in the apices of a chest, etc.). Use a densitometer to measure this area on both the original and duplicated images. Record the OD levels for both. If necessary, repeat the duplication procedure until these levels are within OD 0.30 of one another. (Remember that increased time will decrease density on duplication film and vice versa.)

2. Record the OD level for a light and dark area of both images.

LABORATORY 19-5 (Continued)

Lightening

1. Record on each film the exposure time used.

2. Record the OD levels for the same average density area on each of the films. Record these OD readings on the D log E graph that follows.

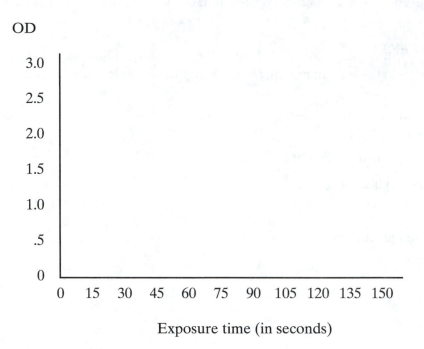

OD

Exposure time (in seconds)

ANALYSIS

Duplication

1. How much difference (in OD #) did you record between the original and duplicated film for the light area? For the average area? For the dark area?

2. Are the two images identical in contrast? If not, why?

Lightening

1. According to the data on your D log E curve, what is the relationship between time and density when using duplicating film?

2. Construct a duplicating exposure time technique chart for lightening images that are too dark.

WORKSHEET 20-1 AUTOMATIC FILM PROCESSING CHEMISTRY

PURPOSE

Identify and critically examine the use and function of the chemicals used in the automatic radiographic film processing cycle.

FOR FURTHER REVIEW

Refer to Chapter 20 in the accompanying textbook for further review of this topic.

ACTIVITIES

Answer the following questions.

1. Briefly describe the principle for the action of film development by filling in the blanks.

   The primary elements of the developer are _____ agents. These agents give up _____, neutralizing the positive ions in the sensitivity specks which make up the latent image. This reduction results in the formation of _____ metallic _____, which transforms the latent image into a _____ image.

2. List the three factors that must be controlled in order for the reduction process to produce the correct radiographic density?

3. What is the major by-product of the reduction process and what are its effects?

4. Match the function of the developer components listed in column A with the chemical action listed in column B. Indicate your answer by placing the correct number in the blank.

   Column A—Function   Column B—Action

   _____ **a.** Solvent   **1.** Serve as electron donors to the latent image site, resulting in the crystal being converted to black metallic silver.

   _____ **b.** Reducing agent/s

   _____ **c.** Activator   **2.** Swells and softens the film's emulsion so the exposed silver halide crystals can be evenly reduced, while maintaining the solution's alkaline state.

   _____ **d.** Restrainer

   _____ **e.** Preservative   **3.** Inhibits the reducing agents so that they only reduce the exposed silver bromide crystals.

   _____ **f.** Hardener

                                        4. Prevents rapid oxidation of the reducing agents.

                                        5. Reduces emulsion swelling.

                                        6. Medium for dissolving the chemicals.

5. Match each automatic processor developer chemical in column B with its correct function or action in column A. Indicate your answer by placing the correct number in the blank.

Column A—Function/Action

_____ **a.** Reduces oxidation

_____ **b.** Controls the activity of reducing agents

_____ **c.** Rapid reduction producing gray shades

_____ **d.** Hardening agent

_____ **e.** Slow reduction producing black shades

_____ **f.** Aids reduction by swelling the emusion

Column B—Chemical

1. Hydroquinone

2. Glutaraldehyde

3. Sodium carbonate

4. Sodium sulfite

5. Potassium bromide

6. Phenidone

6. Why is the fixing step in automatic film processing so important?

7. What is meant by "clearing time"?

8. When cleaning an automatic processor, why is it important to fill the processor's fixer tank before the developer tank?

9. Match the function of the fixer components listed in column A with the chemical action listed in column B. Indicate your answer by placing the correct number in the blank.

Column A—Function

_____ **a.** Solvent

_____ **b.** Clearing agent

_____ **c.** Activator

_____ **d.** Hardener

_____ **e.** Preservative

Column B—Action

1. Maintains the solution's acidic state

2. Stabilizes the emulsion, aiding transport efficiency

3. Removes unexposed silver halide from the emulsion

4. Maintains fixer chemicals in suspension

5. Extends the life of the "hypo"

10. Match each chemical in column B with its correct function or action in column A. Indicate your answer by placing the correct number in the blank. Numbers may be used more than once.

<u>Column A—Function/Action</u>   <u>Column B—Chemical</u>

_____ **a.** Stops development   **1.** Ammonium thiosulfate

_____ **b.** Clearing agent   **2.** Potassium alum

_____ **c.** Preservative   **3.** Acetic acid

_____ **d.** Hardener   **4.** Water

_____ **e.** Solvent   **5.** Sodium sulfite

11. The archiving process in automatic film processing is accomplished by
_____ and _____ the film.

12. The _____ step in automatic processing effectively removes all residual chemicals from the film.

13. List the two factors that expedite the wash cycle in automatic processing.

a.

b.

14. What is the final step in the auto processing cycle?

15. List two functions of the drying step in the automatic processor.

a.

b.

LABORATORY 20-2 FILM PROCESSING TIME AND TEMPERATURE

PURPOSE

Demonstrate the effects of time and temperature on radiographic density and contrast.

FOR FURTHER REVIEW

Refer to Chapter 20 in the accompanying textbook for further review of this topic.

MATERIALS

1. Automatic film processor

2. Sensitometer

3. Photographic thermometer

4. 8″ × 10″ radiographic image receptor

5. Densitometer

PROCEDURES

1. In the darkroom with the white lights off, write the number 1 on a sheet of 8″ × 10″ radiographic film using a lead pencil. Expose the film with a sensitometer.

2. Turn on a processor that has not been running for some time (it is necessary that developer temperature be less than optimal). Immediately process film #1. Record the developer temperature by using the photographic thermometer immersed in the developer tank.

3. Wait for the developer temperature to reach normal operating level. Repeat step 1, but mark the film #2.

4. Develop film #2. Measure and record the temperature of the developer by using a photographic thermometer immersed in the developer tank.

5. Repeat step 1, but mark the film #3.

6. Feed film #3 into the processor. Exactly 10 seconds after the trailing end of the film has entered the processor, turn the processor off for exactly 1 minute. At the end of the 60 seconds, turn the processor back on.

7. Using a densitometer, measure the ODs of the steps for film #2. Locate the step number closest to an OD of 1.2 and identify this step as the speed step. Record the OD measured at the speed step along with the OD of the second step above the speed step in the Results section.

   NOTE: The step # identified as the speed step for film #2 must also be used for films #1 and #3.

8. Use a densitometer to measure the ODs of the assigned speed step and second step above the speed step on films #1 and #3 and record the measurements in the Results section.

LABORATORY 20-2 (Continued)

RESULTS

	Film #1	Film #2	Film #3
OD of speed step # (Density)	_____	_____	_____
OD of second step above speed step	_____	_____	_____
Difference between the two steps (Contrast)	_____	_____	_____

ANALYSIS

1. Assuming that the radiographic density (speed step) and contrast (difference between the two OD measurements) of film #2 represent optimal image quality, summarize the effects that development temperature and time have on radiographic density and contrast.

2. Modern automatic film processors complete the development stage of the film processing sequence in approximately 20 seconds, while manual film processing requires 3 to 5 minutes for the development stage to be completed. Explain why these times are so different.

3. What is the typical developer temperature range used in a modern 90-second radiographic film processor?

4. The two components of the developer solution that are responsible for producing radiographic density on the film work in a synergistic manner. What are these components and explain this process.

5. List two factors that could affect (alter) the developer temperature.

LABORATORY 20-3 AUTOMATIC FILM PROCESSOR

PURPOSE

Identify and critically examine the function of the listed automatic processor parts or systems, processor malfunctions, and recommend appropriate corrective action.

FOR FURTHER REVIEW

Refer to Chapter 20 in the accompanying textbook for further review of this topic.

MATERIALS

1. Automatic film processor

PROCEDURES

The instructor will identify and explain the principle of each of the following:

1. Feed tray
2. Entrance rollers
3. Drive motor system
4. Recirculation system
5. Transport racks
   Developer, fixer, and wash
   turnarounds
6. Crossover networks
   Labels, alignment, and
   guide shoes
7. Dryer tubes
8. Immersion time

9. Water requirements
   Consumption and filters
10. Temperature
    Adjustments
    Heat exchanger
    Dryer temperature
11. Replenishment
    Rate adjustments
    Line filters
    Oxidation covers
12. Standby unit
13. Silver recovery connection

RESULTS

1. Using the following diagram of a modern automatic radiographic film processor, fill in the blanks with the appropriate components.

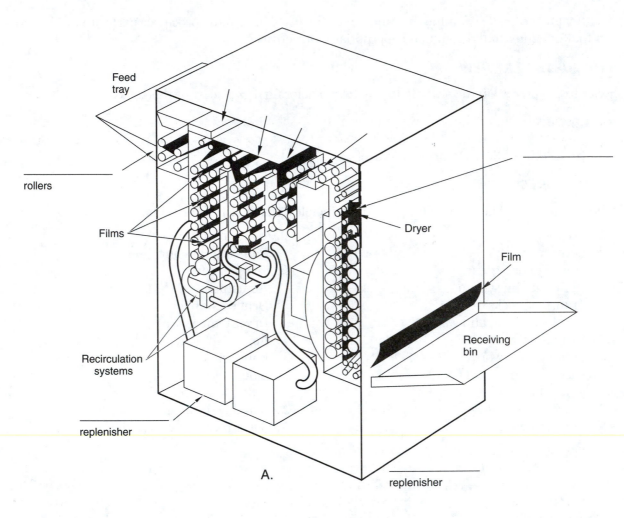

Feed
tray

_____
rollers

Films

Recirculation
systems

_____
replenisher

A.

Dryer

Film

Receiving
bin

_____
replenisher

ANALYSIS

1. What are the functions of the replenishment and recirculation systems? How are they similar? How are they different?

2. Discuss the significance of water temperature as it affects developer temperature. In most processors (noncold water models), what are the common limits of water temperature as related to the desired developer temperature?

3. What is the function of the heat exchanger? Where is one located?

4. Calculate the water saved by using a standby unit. Assume an automatic processor operates 40 hours per week for 52 weeks per year and uses 2 1/2 gallons of water per minute. How many gallons of water would be used during the 1-year period? If you added a standby unit, it would reduce the volume of water used during the nonoperational times of the processor. Assume that during the 40-hour processor work week, the processor is in the standby mode for 5 hours per day. Water use during the 5 hours standby mode is 1 gallon per minute. How many gallons of water are saved over a full year? Be sure to consider the fully operational time and the time spent in standby.

5. What advantages are there to having a standby unit? What are the disadvantages?

6. Explain how you could identify the diameter of a scratched roller from the processed radiograph.

7. How can you determine whether scratches on a radiograph are caused by the guide shoes of a crossover or by the turnaround?

8. In your clinic you have undertaken a recent contract that will greatly increase the number of 8″ × 10″ radiographs processed. What consideration should be given to changing replenishment rates per 14″ × 17″ film if the total number of films per day remains unchanged? Why?

9. List and describe three different types of silver recovery units that are used on automatic radiographic film processors.

LABORATORY 21-1 RADIOGRAPHIC FILM CHARACTERISTICS

PURPOSE

Evaluate film contrast and speed.

FOR FURTHER REVIEW

Refer to Chapters 20 and 21 in the accompanying textbook for further review of this topic.

MATERIALS

1. Automatic film processor

2. Three different types of orthochromatic film

3. Sensitometer

4. Densitometer

5. Graph paper

PROCEDURES

1. Ask your lab instructor for three different radiographic films. In the darkroom, mark one film with the letter A and the others with the letters B and C. These identification letters should be used any time you are describing a particular film.

2. Expose the three films in a sensitometer. Expose one edge of the film, then turn it over and expose the opposite edge of the film. This will expose both sides of the emulsion.

3. Make sure the developer temperature is at the optimal temperature, then process all the films at one time.

4. Use a densitometer to read and record the densities of each of the sensitometric steps on both emulsion sides of each of the three films. In addition obtain the base plus fog level for each film by measuring a cleared area on the film. Average the densities obtained on each side for every step. Use the averaged step density reading.

5. Use graph paper to construct a sensitometric curve for each film. Graph all three films on the same graph with each in a different color.

6. Analyze the sensitometric curves constructed for each film. Record the data necessary to calculate the average gradient (contrast) and relative speed for each film on the film characteristics data form. Remember that net density is the density delivered to the film by the exposure itself (the density above the base plus fog).

7. Use the recorded data to calculate the average gradient (contrast) for each film from a net density of 0.25 to 2.5. Show the calculations and record the solutions on the data form.

LABORATORY 21–1 (Continued)

RESULTS

FILM CHARACTERISTICS DATA FORM

	Film A	Film B	Film C
Base + Fog			
Log Relative Exposure @ Net Density 0.25			
Log Relative Exposure @ Net Density 2.5			
Log Relative Exposure @ Net Density 1.0			
Film Constrast			

CALCULATIONS

LABORATORY 21-1 (Continued)

ANALYSIS

1. What is base plus fog? What impact does it have on film characteristics?

2. Which film exhibited the highest film contrast? The least? How did you calculate the contrast values?

3. What can be said relative to the exposure latitude of the three films? The film latitude?

4. Which film exhibited the highest film speed? The least?

5. Assume that it took 20 mAs to achieve a net density of 1.0 on film A. How much mAs would be required to achieve a net density of 1.0 on Film B? On Film C?

6. What is the relationship between film speed and contrast? Do your data support this?

7. What is the relationship between film latitude and contrast? Do your data support this?

LABORATORY 22-1 INTENSIFYING SCREEN EMISSION SPECTRA

PURPOSE

Demonstrate the color and intensity of light emitted from intensifying screens and evaluate the effect of film and screen spectral emission on film/screen combination speed.

FOR FURTHER REVIEW

Refer to Chapter 22 and Chapter 23 in the accompanying textbook for further review of this topic.

MATERIALS

1. Energized radiographic unit

2. Automatic film processor

3. 2 Blue light-emitting rare-earth cassettes (lanthanum oxybromide) with different RS values

4. 2 Green light-emitting rare-earth cassettes (gandolinium oxysulfide) with different RS values

5. Step wedge (penetrometer)

6. Densitometer

SUGGESTED EXPOSURE FACTORS

Procedure A—70 kVp, 50mA, 2 sec (this may not be possible with an mAs unit, but choose the longest exposure time possible)

Procedure B—60 kVp, 20mAs, 40″ SID, nongrid

PROCEDURE A

1. Unload the film from the four cassettes, if necessary. Open the cassettes and place them on the tabletop so a corner of each of the four open cassettes is common to the others.

2. Note the RS and rare-earth phosphor material of each of the different cassettes.

3. Using a 40″ SID, center the x-ray tube to the point where all four corners meet and open the collimator as wide as possible to include as much of each of the four cassettes as possible.

4. Turn off the room lights and observe the screen fluorescent through the viewing window of the control booth while making an exposure.

PROCEDURE B

1. Choose two cassettes with the same RS but different rare-earth phosphors and load both cassettes with the same type of film. Note whether your particular film is blue sensitive or green sensitive.

2. Place one cassette on the radiographic table and center the step wedge on the cassette so that it is perpendicular to the anode-cathode axis of the x-ray tube, placing the thicker end of the penetrometer at the cathode end of the x-ray tube.

LABORATORY 22-1 (Continued)

3. Collimate the x-ray beam to the step wedge exposure the radiograph, identify the cassette, and process the film.

4. Repeat steps 2 and 3 with the second cassette.

5. Use a densitometer to measure the optical densities (OD) of the steps on each of the radiographs and record them on the appropriate data form.

6. Use the densitometer to record the base + fog level of each radiograph. Subtract the base + fog value from the OD readings for each film and record the results (net OD) in the data form.

RESULTS

SPECTRAL EMISSION AND INTENSITY

Phosphor Material	RS	Color	Light Intensity

SPECTRAL MATCHING AND SENSITIVITY DATA FORM

Film Sensitivity				
Screen Emission	Blue		Green	
Step Number	OD	Net OD	OD	Net OD
1				
2				
3				
4				
5				
6				
7				
8				
9				
10				

LABORATORY 22-1 (Continued)

ANALYSIS

1. Describe the intensity (brightness) of the light given off by the four cassettes. Does there appear to be any correlation between the light intensity and the speed of the screens exposed? Explain.

2. Describe the color(s) of the light emitted by the screens. Does there appear to be any correlation between the color of light emitted and the screen phosphor type? Explain.

3. Is there a speed difference between the images obtained with and without correct spectral matching of the radiographic film and intensifying screen? Explain.

4. Do you feel that the speed difference is significant? Why?

LABORATORY 23-1 EVALUATING RADIOGRAPHIC FILM/SCREEN COMBINATIONS

PURPOSE

Determine appropriate film/screen combinations for various clinical situations, formulate basic technical factors, and approximate exposure for various film/screen combinations.

FOR FURTHER REVIEW

Refer to Chapter 23 in the accompanying textbook for further review of this topic.

MATERIALS

1. Energized radiographic unit

2. Densitometer

3. Automatic film processor

4. Various different intensifying screens in cassettes

5. Various films compatible with the screens

6. Radiographic phantom (e.g., skull or knee)

7. Resolution test tool

8. Step wedge (penetrometer) with marker or dot on a middle step

9. Dosimeter (digital ion chamber recommended)

SUGGESTED EXPOSURE FACTORS

RS (see the procedure), 30 mAs, 65 kVp, 40″ SID, nongrid
The mA station must not vary between exposures (100 mA recommended).

PROCEDURES

1. Expose a control film of the following items with a single exposure:

> phantom in lateral position
> resolution tool (under phantom)
> aluminum step wedge (next to phantom)
> dosimeter ion chamber

The marked step of the step wedge must exhibit an optical density (OD) of 1.30 to 1.70. If necessary, adjust the exposure factors and repeat until the OD standard has been achieved. Time changes are recommended although kVp can be modified if necessary to achieve the OD range. Record the OD of the marked step and the dose reading in mR and then develop normally.

2. Repeat step 1 using at least one other film and one other set of intensifying screens until at least four different film/screen combinations have been produced.

LABORATORY 23-1 (Continued)

RESULTS

1. Complete the data in the following table.

Combination		mAs	OD	lp/mm	mR
Film	Screen				

ANALYSIS

1. Rank the film/screen combinations according to the mAs required to produce similar densities on the film. Why did you need to use different mAs for different film/screen combinations?

2. Rank the film/screen combinations according to approximate exposure dose that a patient would have received (use your mAs ratings). Describe any correlation between mAs and exposure.

3. Using the lp/mm rankings, describe any correlation between the mAs and the resolving power of the system. Describe any relationship between the resolution and exposure.

LABORATORY 23-1 (Continued)

4. Recommend film/screen combinations for each of the following clinical situations when maximum resolution is required. Use good judgment on contrast, latitude, and exposure.

   a. portable chest radiography

   b. general emergency room radiography

   c. newborn intensive care unit abdominal radiography

   d. navicular wrist magnification radiography

5. Repeat step 4 with patient exposure as the primary requirement.

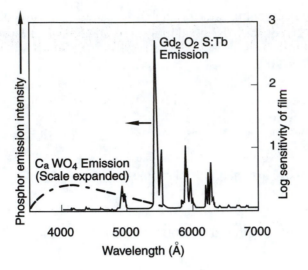

6. Draw in an approximate curve for blue sensitive film and another curve for green sensitive film on the preceding graph. Below what wavelength would both films produce an image? Above what wavelength would only the green sensitive film produce an image?

WORKSHEET 24-1 DIGITAL IMAGE PROCESSING

PURPOSE

Describe the process of digital image data acquisition and reconstruction.

FOR FURTHER REVIEW

Refer to Chapter 24 in the accompanying textbook for further review of this topic.

ACTIVITIES

1. If density measurements of the pixels in Figure A were made, they might be expressed as the numbers shown in Figure B. This is essentially a digitization of the information shown in Figure A.

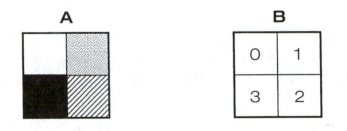

2. If the box is irradiated, the attenuation data received for various projections by adding the density values for each line of values within the pixels would appear as follows:

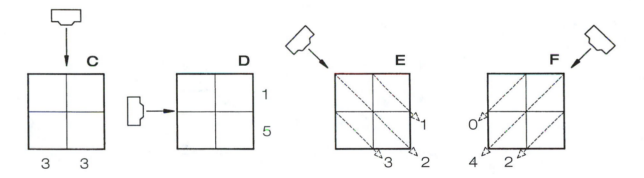

3. A computed tomography unit accumulates information in a much more complex, but similar, process. When considering only a single projection, the computer assumes that the density values for each pixel are equal as shown in Figure G.

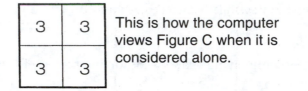

This is how the computer views Figure C when it is considered alone.

Because this is obviously not accurate, it is necessary to develop a method for the computer to compare and weigh the information from each projection to obtain an accurate image.

4. To reconstruct the information in Figure B, which would then permit the image in Figure A to be created, the computer must backproject the attenuation data received for the various projections (Figures C, D, E, and F).

Using only the information given in Figures C, D, E, and F, total the attenuation for each pixel by summing the accumulated total for each projection as shown in Figure H.

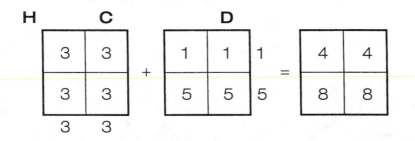

Use Figure I to continue to add the pixel attenuation data from Figures E and F.

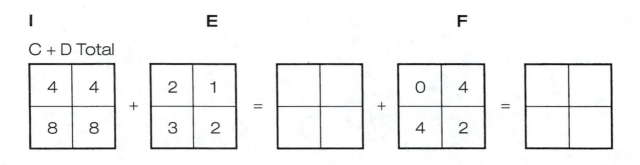

5. The information in Figure I can then be manipulated mathematically to reconstruct Figure B. First subtract the background value (the minimum number for any pixel), which is 6.

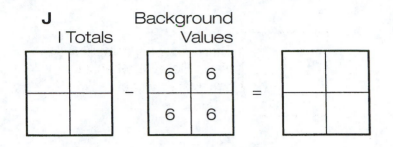

J
I Totals   Background Values

Then divide each pixel by 3 to reconstruct Figure B. This number is achieved in computed tomography by complex formulas based on many variables within the system.

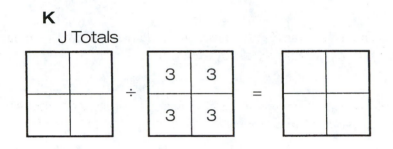

K
J Totals

LABORATORY 24-2 CONTROLLING AND EVALUATING DIGITAL IMAGES

PURPOSE

Explain the function of digital image window level and width controls.

FOR FURTHER REVIEW

Refer to Chapter 24 in the accompanying textbook for further review of this topic.

MATERIALS

1. Computed tomography or magnetic resonance imaging console

PROCEDURE

1. Request a technologist who is familiar with the operating console to bring up an average image and adjust it to diagnostic window levels. Have the technologist indicate which controls operate the image window level and width. Also have this technologist indicate which numbers on the monitor indicate the window level and width. Record these numbers for use during this laboratory.

2. Use only the window level control to make the image completely light. Record this number. Carefully observe the effect on the demonstration of various structures as the window level is slowly increased to complete darkness. Record this number. Bring the window level back to the original number. Watch the monitor closely while the window level is very slowly increased. Record the number when the first visible change is observed.

3. Use only the window width control to make the image completely light. Record this number. Carefully observe the effect on the demonstration of various structures as the window width is slowly increased to complete darkness. Record this number. Bring the window width back to the original number. Watch the monitor closely while the window width is very slowly increased. Record the number when the first visible change is observed.

RESULTS

1. Record the window level and width numbers as indicated in the preceding procedures.

2. Subtract the window level number for the light image from the dark image and record the result as the range (R). Subtract the window level number for the light image from the original diagnostic quality image and record the result as the diagnostic level (D). Use the formula D/R $\times$ 100 to determine the percentage of window level that produced the diagnostic image.

3. Repeat this process for the window width numbers.

LABORATORY 24–2 (Continued)

ANALYSIS

1. What visible image quality factor is changing as the window level is varied?

2. What visible image quality factor is changing as the window width is varied?

3. Which primary mathematical functions is the computer applying to the image pixel data as the window level is changed?

4. Which primary mathematical functions is the computer applying to the image pixel data as the window width is changed?

5. What percentage change was required to see a density change?

6. What percentage change was required to see a contrast change?

7. What percent of the total available range of density produced the diagnostic quality image?

8. What percent of the total available range of contrast produced the diagnostic quality image?

LABORATORY 25-1 COMPUTED RADIOGRAPHY

PURPOSE

Investigate the exposure latitude characteristics of a given CR system.

FOR FURTHER REVIEW

Refer to Chapter 25 in the accompanying textbook for further review of this topic.

MATERIALS

1. CR imaging system

2. Automatic film processor

3. Phantom body part

4. Radiographic film with cassettes

PROCEDURE A   ANALOG EXPOSURE RANGE BASELINE

1. Using a radiographic film screen combination produce a diagnostic quality image of a phantom body part.

2. Produce four additional images using 1/4, 1/2, 2×, and 4× (the mAs value utilized in the previous step).

3. Produce four additional images using –30 percent, –15 percent, +15 percent, and +30 percent of the kVp value utilized in step 1.

PROCEDURE B   CR EXPOSURE COMPENSATION LIMITS FOR mAs

1. Repeat procedures A1 and A2 using a CR system and an appropriate exposure procedure for the phantom part.

PROCEDURE C   CR EXPOSURE COMPENSATION LIMITS FOR kVp

1. Repeat procedures A1 and A3 using a CR system and an appropriate exposure procedure for the phantom part.

RESULTS

Using the images produced in Procedure A as the baseline for comparison, review the images produced in Procedures B and C in respect to image quality.

ANALYSIS

1. Considering the set of images produced in Procedures A, B, and C, which would you be willing to submit for diagnosis?

2. What is your assessment of the CR compensation range for insufficient and excessive mAs?

3. What is your assessment of the CR compensation range for insufficient and excessive kVp?

4. In reviewing the images in Procedures B and C, are you able to detect a difference in the level of noise present in the images? How would you account for this?

5. What recommendations can you make for this CR system for setting technical factors? Be sure you include both high and low ranges as well as specify how close factors must be to an appropriate manual exposure technique to produce acceptable quality CR images.

LABORATORY 25-2 COMPUTED RADIOGRAPHIC PROCESSING ERRORS

PURPOSE

Demonstrate the effect of common errors in obtaining and processing computed radiographic images.

FOR FURTHER REVIEW

Refer to Chapter 25 in the accompanying textbook for further review of this topic.

MATERIALS

1. Energized radiographic unit

2. 5 8″ × 10″ or 10″ × 12″ CR cassettes

3. 18″ × 10″ or 10″ × 12″ film/screen cassette

4. Wrist phantom

5. Automatic film processor

SUGGESTED EXPOSURE FACTORS

50 kVp, 5 mAs, nongrid tabletop, 40″ SID

PROCEDURES

1. Erase all CR cassettes before beginning this laboratory to ensure they are clean.

2. Place a CR cassette on top of a radiographic table. Center the wrist phantom to the middle of the cassette and center the CR for a proper wrist image. Collimate the beam so that there is at least a 25-inch collimated border on all four sides of the image.

3. Place second CR cassette and the film/screen on the tabletop approximately 1 foot from the cassette being used to image the wrist. These cassettes should remain on the tabletop for all four exposures, but NOT be exposed to the primary x-ray beam. They will be used to evaluate the CR system's sensitivity to scatter radiation.

4. Expose the wrist image and process the image using the correct algorithm for a PA wrist image. Label this image as "#1, baseline image." Evaluate this image and record the exposure index.

5. Repeat step 1, but process the image using an abdomen algorithm. Label this image as "#2, histogram error." Evaluate the image and record the exposure index.

6. Repeat step 1, placing the write phantom off-center to the left of the cassette. Collimate the beam so that there is at least a 2-inch collimated border on all four sides of the image.

7. Expose the wrist image and process the image using the correct algorithm for a PA wrist image. Label this image as "#3, off-center error." Evaluate the image and record the exposure index.

8. Repeat step 1, placing the wrist phantom off-center to the left of the cassette. Adjust the collimator so that the radiation field extends beyond the left side, top and bottom of the cassette (only the right side should have a crisp collimated border).

9. Expose the wrist image and process the image using the correct algorithm for a PA wrist image. Label this image as "#4, collimator edge identification error." Evaluate the image and record the exposure index.

10. Process the CR cassette left on the tabletop for the three exposures using the algorithm for a PA wrist image. Mark this image as "#5, CR scatter sensitivity." Evaluate the image and record the exposure index.

11. Process the film/screen cassette left on the tabletop for the three exposures in the automatic film processor. Label this image as "#6, film/screen scatter sensitivity." Evaluate the image.

RESULTS

1. Compare image #1 and image #2.

   a. What effect is seen as a result of the histogram error?

   b. What is the basis for the difference in the two images?

   c. Are both images of diagnostic quality?

   d. Are the exposure indices different? Why or why not?

2. Compare image #1 and image #3.

   a. What effect is seen as a result of the off-center positioning error?

   b. What is the basis for the difference in the two images?

   c. Are both images of diagnostic quality?

   d. Are the exposure indices different? Why or why not?

3. Compare image #1 and image #4.

   a. What effect is seen as a result of the collimator edge index error?

   b. What is the basis for the difference in the two images?

   c. Are both images of diagnostic quality?

   d. Are the exposure indices different? Why or why not?

4. Compare image #5 and image #6.

   a. What effect is seen as a result of the scatter radiation on each image?

   b. What is the basis for the difference in the two images?

5. Of the four errors made in utilizing the CR system, which error most greatly affected the image quality?

WORKSHEET 26–1 DIGITAL IMAGE MANAGEMENT

PURPOSE
Explain the purpose of managing digital information in an imaging department.

FOR FURTHER REVIEW
Refer to Chapter 26 in the accompanying textbook for further review of this topic.

ACTIVITIES

1. Specify three advantages of digital imaging management in comparison to traditional film/screen environments.

2. What is network infrastructure and how does it impact on image and information distribution?

3. What formula is used to calculate digital image size? Why is this important? Which digital images are largest in size: CT, MR, or digital radiographs?

4. What is the difference between a LAN and a WAN? How is each used in an imaging department?

5. What type of CRT monitors is used by referring physicians for soft-copy display? Are different monitors required by radiologists and QC technologies? Why or why not?

6. What are the advantages to using LCD monitors for soft-copy display instead of a CRT?

7. What does the acronym DICOM stand for and why is it important in digital image management?

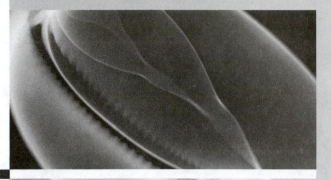

UNIT IV Analyzing the Image

LABORATORY 27-1 EVALUATING ACCEPTANCE LIMITS

PURPOSE

Determine the approximate diagnostic image quality acceptance limits for screen/film receptors and digital radiographic systems.

FOR FURTHER REVIEW

Refer to Chapter 27 in the accompanying textbook for further review of this topic.

MATERIALS

1. Energized radiographic unit

2. 14″ × 17″ screen/film cassettes 400 RS

3. 14″ × 17″ CR cassettes or a DR unit

4. Abdomen or pelvis phantom

5. Automatic film processor

6. CR image processor

SUGGESTED EXPOSURE FACTORS

First exposure: 80 kVp, 2.5 mAs, 40″ SID, grid

PROCEDURES

1. Position the abdomen phantom for an AP projection using a screen/film cassette. Center and collimate the beam to the cassette. Expose the cassette and process the film.

2. Repeat step 1 to produce a series of phantom images by increasing the exposure by 2 × mAs increments (5 mAs, 10 mAs, 40 mAs, 80 mAs, 160 mAs). Process the films and clearly number the images with the corresponding mAs values.

3. Repeat steps 1 and 2 using a digital imaging receptor. Process the images using an AP abdomen algorithm and clearly number the images with the corresponding mAs values.

RESULTS

1. Arrange the entire screen/film series on view boxes in order of increasing mAs. If the digital images are printed to film, also arrange them on view boxes in order of increasing mAs. If the digital images are viewed on a monitor, sequence the images for viewing from lowest mAs to highest mAs.

2. Survey as many radiologists, radiographers, and students as possible. Ask each professional to record only those images that are unacceptable for diagnosis in each set of images. The goal is to determine which images from each set could be submitted for diagnosis, not which is the best image.

3. Create two subsets of histogram graphs (x-axis = mAs value, y-axis = number of respondents submitting image for diagnosis) by drawing vertical bars to indicate how many persons said they would submit each image for diagnosis. The subset should be created as follows:

   a. Screen/film images
      i. Radiologists
      ii. Radiographers
      iii. Students
   b. Digital images
      i. Radiologists
      ii. Radiographers
      iii. Students

ANALYSIS

1. Compare the histograms for each subset and discuss why the groups are similar or different.

2. Compare the histograms for the same population, but comparing screen/film images to digital images, and discuss the differences and similarities.

3. Compare your personal opinion of the images in both sets to the results you obtained for each group. Explain the possible reasons for all differences.

4. How do the acceptable ranges vary from screen/film to digital receptors?

5. According to your data, which system exhibits the widest latitude? Explain your answer.

6. List the advantages and disadvantages to utilizing an image receptor with a wide latitude.

LABORATORY 28-1 THE EFFECT OF mAs ON DENSITY

PURPOSE

Demonstrate the effect of mAs on image density for screen/film receptors.

FOR FURTHER REVIEW

Refer to Chapter 28 in the accompanying textbook for further review of this topic.

MATERIALS

1. Energized radiographic unit

2. 10″ × 12″ screen/film cassettes 100 RS

3. Wrist phantom

4. Step wedge

5. Automatic film processor

6. Densitometer

SUGGESTED EXPOSURE FACTORS

First exposure: 60 kVp, 2.5 mAs, 40″ SID, nongrid

PROCEDURES

Part A

1. Place a 10″ × 12″ screen/film cassette crosswise on top of the radiographic table. Using lead masks, divide the cassette into thirds in a crosswise fashion to obtain three exposures on one film.

2. Center the wrist phantom and step wedge on the unmasked portion. Label this image "A." Center and collimate the beam to the unmasked portion of the film. Expose the cassette.

3. Rearrange the masks and place the phantom in the middle section of the cassette. Center and collimate the beam to the unmasked portion of the film. Expose the cassette using 60 kVp, 5 mAs, 40″ SID.

4. Rearrange the masks and place the phantom in the final third of the cassette. Center and collimate the beam to the unmasked portion of the film. Expose the cassette using 60 kVp, 10 mAs, 40″ SID. Process the film.

5. Using a densitometer, measure and record the OD of step 6 on the step wedge images.

Part B (Only if you have radiographic unit that allows the operator to choose mA and time separately)

1. Place a 10″ × 12″ screen/film cassette crosswise on top of the radiographic table. Using lead masks, divide the cassette into thirds in a crosswise fashion to obtain three exposures on one film.

2. Center the wrist phantom and step wedge on the unmasked portion. Label this image "B." Center and collimate the beam to the unmasked portion of the film. Expose the cassette using 60 kVp, 50 mA, 1/10 sec, and 40″ SID.

LABORATORY 28-1 (Continued)

3. Rearrange the masks and place the phantom in the middle section of the cassette. Center and collimate the beam to the unmasked portion of the film. Expose the cassette using 60 kVp, 100 mA, 1/20 sec, 40″ SID.

4. Rearrange the masks and place the phantom in the final third of the cassette. Center and collimate the beam to the unmasked portion of the film. Expose the cassette using 60 kVp, 200 mA, 1/40 sec, 40″ SID. Process the film.

5. Using a densitometer, measure and record the OD of step 6 on the step wedge images.

RESULTS

Image A	2.5 mAs	5 mAs	10 mAs
OD step 6			

Image B	50 mAs, 1/10 s	100 mA, 1/20 s	200 mA, 1/40 s
OD step 6			

ANALYSIS

1. What is the effect observed on the radiographic density of each of the three images in part A as the mAs is increased?

2. What is the physical basis for the occurrence of these changes?

3. Do these results prove the theory proposed in Chapter 28 of the textbook? Why or why not?

4. What is the effect observed on the radiographic density of each of the three images in part B?

5. What is the physical basis for this occurrence?

6. What law is supported or not supported by the results part B?

7. Do you think your results would be the same if you repeated both parts A and B, but measured the exposure with a densitometer instead of measuring optical density of a screen/film image receptor? Why or why not?

Name _____ Course _____ Date _____

LABORATORY 28-2 THE EFFECT OF kVp ON DENSITY— THE 15 PERCENT RULE

PURPOSE

Demonstrate the effects of kilovoltage on exposure/film density and the control of radiographic density by changing kVp and mAs utilizing the 15 percent rule.

FOR FURTHER REVIEW

Refer to Chapter 28 in the accompanying textbook for further review of this topic.

MATERIALS

1. Energized radiographic unit
2. Automatic film processor
3. 14″ × 17″ cassette and image receptor
4. Knee phantom
5. Step wedge
6. Densitometer

SUGGESTED EXPOSURE FACTORS

400 RS, see procedure for mA, sec, and kVp, 40″ SID, nongrid

PROCEDURES

A. kVp versus Density

1. Place a 14″ × 17″ cassette crosswise on top of the radiographic table. Using lead masks, divide the cassette into thirds in a crosswise fashion for three exposures on one receptor.
2. Center the phantom knee and step wedge on the unmasked portion. Label the film A, center the central ray, and collimate the beam to the unmasked portion of the receptor. Make an exposure at 75 kVp, 2 mAs, and 40″ SID.
3. Rearrange the masks to reveal the middle third of the cassette and repeat step 2. Change the kVp to 65 and expose the image receptor.
4. Rearrange the masks to reveal the final third of the cassette and repeat step 2. Change the kVp to 86 and expose the image receptor.
5. Process film A.
6. Using a densitometer, measure and record the OD of step 6 of the step wedge images.

B. 15 Percent Rule for Density Control

1. Place a 14″ × 17″ cassette crosswise on top of the radiographic table. Using lead masks, divide the cassette into thirds in a crosswise fashion for three exposures on one image receptor.
2. Center the phantom knee and step wedge on the unmasked portion. Label the receptor, center the central ray, and collimate the beam to the unmasked portion of the receptor. Make an exposure at 75 kVp, 2 mAs, and 40″ SID.
3. Rearrange the masks to reveal the middle third of the cassette and repeat step 2. Decrease the kVp to 65 and, using the 15 percent rule, calculate the mAs to be used with the new kVp and expose the receptor.

LABORATORY 28-2 (Continued)

4. Rearrange the masks to reveal the final third of the cassette and repeat step 2. Increase the kVp to 86 and, using the 15 percent rule, calculate the mAs to be used with the new kVp and expose the receptor.

5. Process film B.

6. Using a densitometer, measure and record the OD of step 6 of the step wedge images.

RESULTS

	OD step 6		
	75 kV	65 kV	86 kV
Image A	_____	_____	_____
Image B	_____	_____	_____

ANALYSIS

1. Discuss the density of the three images in procedure A using both visual and quantitative data.

2. Discuss the density of the three images in procedure B using both visual and quantitative data.

3. How do the visual and quantitative results in procedure B compare with the images obtained with similar kVp used in procedure A? Explain.

4. What is the theory behind the results in procedure B? Do your results support the theory? Explain.

5. What observations can you make about the contrast of the three images in procedure B? In procedure A?

LABORATORY 28-3 DETERMINING ADEQUATE PENETRATION

PURPOSE

Demonstrate the effects of x-ray penetration in regard to adequate demonstration of the visibility of the object imaged using both screen/film and digital radiographic receptors.

FOR FURTHER REVIEW

Refer to Chapter 28 in the accompanying textbook for further review of this topic.

MATERIALS

1. Energized radiographic unit

2. Skull phantom

3. Automatic film processor

4. CR image processor

5. 10″ × 12″ 400 RS screen/film cassettes and film

6. 10″ × 12″ CR cassettes

7. Densitometer

SUGGESTED EXPOSURE FACTORS

Initial exposure: 80 kVp, 10 mAs, 40″ SID, 8:1 Bucky grid

PROCEDURES

1. Place a 400 RS cassette in the Bucky tray and position the phantom on the tabletop for a lateral skull, with the central ray centered to the sella turcica. Collimate to the cassette size, and expose and process the film. Label this film as #1.

2. Repeat step 1, but reduce the kVp to 40 and increase the mAs to 100. Expose and process the film. Label this film as #2.

3. Repeat step 2, but increase the mAs to 400. Expose and process the film. Label this film as #3.

4. Repeat steps 1, 2, and 3 using CR cassettes and label the images #4, #5, and #6.

RESULTS

1. Review the three screen/film images side by side, comparing the images for visibility of the petrous portion of the temporal bone and for adequate radiographic density.

2. If possible, print the three CR images to film and review them side by side, comparing the images for visibility of the petrous portion of the temporal bone and for adequate radiographic density. If this is not possible, view the images on a high-resolution monitor to make the comparison.

LABORATORY 28-3 (Continued)

3. Using a densitometer, record the OD density readings in the parietal bone region of the skull and in the petrous portion of the skull for both sets of images.

Image	OD Parietal Bone	OD Petrous Portion	Within Useful OD Range?
1			
2			
3			
4			
5			
6			

ANALYSIS

1. Do the OD readings on any of the images fall within the useful OD range?

2. Which images demonstrate the achievement of satisfactory density and optimal visibility of the petrous portion of the temporal bone? Why?

3. Would satisfactory density of the area of interest be achieved if the mAs was increased to 800 or 1,000? Explain.

4. Describe differences between the screen/film and CR images. Explain the rationale for these differences.

LABORATORY 28-4 THE EFFECT OF DISTANCE ON DENSITY— THE EXPOSURE MAINTENANCE FORMULA

PURPOSE

Demonstrate the effect of SID on radiographic density and the use of the exposure maintenance formula to control exposure/film density.

FOR FURTHER REVIEW

Refer to Chapter 28 in the accompanying textbook for further review of this topic.

MATERIALS

1. Energized radiographic unit
2. Automatic film processor
3. 14″ × 17″ radiographic cassettes and film
4. Knee phantom
5. Step wedge (penetrometer)
6. Densitometer

SUGGESTED EXPOSURE FACTORS

400 RS, see procedure for mA, sec, and kVp, 40″ SID, nongrid

PROCEDURES

Distance and Density

1. Place a 14″ × 17″ cassette crosswise on top of the radiographic table. Using lead masks, divide the cassette into thirds in a crosswise fashion for three exposures on one film.

2. Center the knee phantom and step wedge on the unmasked portion. Label the film "A," center the central ray, and collimate the beam to the unmasked portion of the film. Select 75 kVp, 2 mAs, and 40″ SID, and expose the film.

3. Rearrange the masks to reveal the middle third of the cassette and repeat step 2. Adjust the SID to 60″ and expose the film.

4. Rearrange the masks to reveal the final third of the cassette and repeat step 2. Adjust the SID to 20″, expose the film, and process it.

5. Use a densitometer to measure and record the OD of step 6 of the step wedge.

Exposure Maintenance Formula

1. Place a 14″ × 17″ cassette crosswise on top of the radiographic table. Using lead masks, divide the cassette into thirds in a crosswise fashion for three exposures on one film.

2. Center the knee phantom and step wedge on unmasked portion. Label the film "B," center the central ray, and collimate the beam to the unmasked portion of the film. Select 75 kVp, 2 mAs, and 40″ SID, and expose the film.

LABORATORY 28–4 (Continued)

3. Rearrange the masks to reveal the middle third of the cassette and repeat step 2. Increase the SID to 60″ and, using the exposure maintenance formula, calculate the mAs to be used with the new distance to maintain the density and expose the film.

4. Rearrange the masks to reveal the final third of the cassette and repeat step 2. Decrease the SID to 20″ and, using the exposure maintenance formula, calculate the mAs to be used with the new distance, expose, and process the film.

5. Use a densitometer to measure and record the OD of step 6 of the step wedge.

RESULTS

	OD step 6		
	40″	60″	20″
Image A	_____	_____	_____
Image B	_____	_____	_____

ANALYSIS

1. As the SID is increased, what effect is seen in the density of each of the three images on image A?

2. What is the physical basis for the changes seen on image A?

3. What effect does the manipulation of mAs have on exposure/film density (image B)?

4. What is the physical basis for the results demonstrated on image B?

5. Briefly describe the practical importance of the mAs/distance relationships as seen on image B.

LABORATORY 28-5 THE EFFECT OF FILM/SCREEN COMBINATIONS ON DENSITY

PURPOSE

Demonstrate the effect of different radiographic film/screen combinations on radiographic density.

FOR FURTHER REVIEW

Refer to Chapter 28 in the accompanying textbook for further review of this topic.

MATERIALS

1. Energized radiographic unit

2. Automatic film processor

3. Various speed cassettes

4. Knee phantom

5. Densitometer

6. Step wedge (penetrometer)

SUGGESTED EXPOSURE FACTORS

See procedure for RS, 100 mA, 0.05 sec, 70 kVp, 40″ SID, nongrid

PROCEDURES

1. Produce an image of the knee phantom and step wedge with each of the following film/screen combinations that are available. Use the same exposure factors for each, with the central ray centered and perpendicular to the knee, the step wedge parallel to the knee, and the beam collimated to the cassette size.

   a. Detail (100 RS)   c. Regular (400 RS)

   b. Medium (250 RS)   d. Fast (800 RS)

2. Use a densitometer to record the OD of the middle step (step 6) of each of the four step wedge images.

RESULTS

	OD step 6
Detail	_____
Medium	_____
Regular	_____
Fast	_____

LABORATORY 28-5 (Continued)

ANALYSIS

1. What inferences can be made from the differences in the densities on each of the images?

2. Did the densities appear to follow a uniform progression? Explain.

3. What physical factors dictate the speed (sensitivity) of an intensifying screen?

4. How do screen manufacturers vary the speed of intensifying screens during their construction?

5. What is the purpose of having such a wide variety of screen speeds available?

LABORATORY 28-6 THE EFFECT OF SUBJECT DENSITY AND CONTRAST ON DENSITY

PURPOSE

Demonstrate the effect of different subject densities and contrast on radiographic density.

FOR FURTHER REVIEW

Refer to Chapter 28 in the accompanying textbook for further review of this topic.

MATERIALS

1. Energized radiographic unit

2. Automatic film processor

3. 8″ × 10″ radiographic cassettes with image receptor

4. Shallow container (about 3″ to 4″ deep)

5. Ice cubes

6. 35 mm film canister

7. Super ball 1″ diameter

8. Barium solution

SUGGESTED EXPOSURE FACTORS

100 RS, see procedure for mAs and kVp, 40″ SID, nongrid

PROCEDURES

NOTE: The films produced for this laboratory are also used for Laboratory 29-3, The Effect of Subject Density and Contrast on Image Contrast.

Subject Density and Radiographic Density

1. Fill the container with enough ice cubes to form a single layer. Add water to equal the height of the ice cubes.

2. Mask a cassette in half, center the container to the unmasked portion, collimate, label image #1 and expose at 45 kVp, 1.25 mAs, and 40″ SID.

3. Add water to increase the depth to 2″ in the container. Use the other half of the cassette to repeat steps 2 and 3 and process the receptor.

Subject Contrast and Radiographic Density

1. Place a super ball in an empty 35 mm film canister. Fill the canister with water and replace the cap. Fill the shallow container with water to a depth of 3″ and add the film canister.

2. Mask a cassette in quarters, center the container to an unmasked portion, collimate, label image #2, and expose at 70 kVp, 8 mAs, and 40″ SID.

3. Remove the water from the film canister and replace the super ball and cap. Place the film canister in the shallow container, change the mask, and repeat step 2.

LABORATORY 28-6 (Continued)

4. Fill the film canister with a liquid barium suspension, replace the super ball and the cap to the film canister. Place the film canister in the shallow container. Change the mask and repeat step 2.

5. Remove the barium from the film canister, rinse well with water, replace the super ball in the empty film canister, and replace the cap. Change the mask and center the film canister directly to an unmasked quarter of the cassette (do not place the film canister in the shallow container). Center, collimate, and expose using 70 kVp, 1 mAs, and 40″ SID.

6. Process the film.

RESULTS

1. Review the images on both radiographs for radiographic density.

ANALYSIS

1. What caused the different densities seen in image #1?

2. Why are fewer densities seen in the second exposure on image #1?

3. Which image demonstrates the greatest number of densities on image #2? Why?

4. Which image demonstrates the least number of densities on image #2? Why?

5. Assuming the super ball is a solid tumor, which of the first three images demonstrates its density the best? Why?

LABORATORY 29-1 THE EFFECT OF kVp ON IMAGE CONTRAST

PURPOSE

Demonstrate the effects of kVp on image contrast.

FOR FURTHER REVIEW

Refer to Chapter 29 in the accompanying textbook for further review of this topic.

MATERIALS

1. Energized radiographic unit
2. Automatic film processor
3. 10″ × 12″ cassette with image receptor
4. Step wedge
5. Skull phantom
6. Densitometer

SUGGESTED EXPOSURE FACTORS

400 RS, 100 mA, 0.33 sec, 60 kVp, 40″ SID, 8:1 Bucky grid

PROCEDURES

1. Use a 10″ × 12″ cassette to produce a lateral skull with a step wedge adjacent to it.

2. Use a densitometer to record the OD of steps 4, 5, and 6 of the step wedge. If the OD of step 5 is not 1.2 ± 0.2, adjust the mAs and reexpose.

3. Repeat steps 1 and 2 using 80 kVp, 15 mAs, and 40″ SID.

4. Repeat steps 1 and 2 using 96 kVp, 7.5 mAs, and 40″ SID.

RESULTS

1. Record the OD of steps 4, 5, and 6 below.

2. Calculate the image contrast of each image by subtracting the OD of step 6 from the OD of step 4.

kVp	Step Wedge Optical Density			Contrast
	Step 4	Step 5	Step 6	Step 4 through Step 6
60	_____	_____	_____	_____
80	_____	_____	_____	_____
96	_____	_____	_____	_____

LABORATORY 29-1 (Continued)

ANALYSIS

1. Compare the overall radiographic density of each image individually and then compare the overall densities between the images. Describe your observations. Do your data support your findings? Explain.

2. Describe the observed differences in the contrast between the three images. Explain the reason for the results. Do your data support your observations? Explain.

3. Why do you think it would be advantageous to be able to change the contrast of an image?

4. Define *image contrast*.

5. Explain the difference between long-scale contrast and short-scale contrast.

LABORATORY 29-2 THE EFFECT OF FILM/SCREEN COMBINATIONS ON IMAGE CONTRAST

PURPOSE

Demonstrate the effect that different screen speeds have on image contrast.

FOR FURTHER REVIEW

Refer to Chapter 29 in the accompanying textbook for further review of this topic.

MATERIALS

1. Energized radiographic unit

2. Automatic film processor

3. Various speed cassettes of same phosphor type with same image receptor type

4. Step wedge (penetrometer)

5. Densitometer

SUGGESTED EXPOSURE FACTORS

See procedure.

PROCEDURES

1. Center a cassette on the tabletop. Position the step wedge on the cassette so it is perpendicular to the anode-cathode axis of the x-ray tube.

2. Make the exposures as suggested in the following or as otherwise given by your instructor. Make sure the receptor is permanently identified as to the speed of the screens. Repeat this procedure for each of the remaining film/screen systems and process images.

Screen Type	Relative Speed	Step Wedge Exposure Factors
Fine	100	75 kVp, 25 mA, 1/15 sec
Regular	400	75 kVp, 25 mA, 1/40 sec
Fast	800	75 kVp, 25 mA, 1/60 sec

3. Using a densitometer, measure the OD (optical density) of steps 4, 5, and 6 on the penetrometer for all the radiographs. Record the OD readings. The OD of step 5 should be 1.2 ± 0.2 for all four images. If not, adjust the mAs and reexpose.

LABORATORY 29-2 (Continued)

RESULTS

1. Record the optical density measurements of steps 4, 5, and 6 in the following.

2. Calculate the image contrast of each image by subtracting the OD of step 6 from the OD of step 4.

Screen	RS	Step Wedge Optical Density			Contrast
		Step 4	Step 5	Step 6	Step 4 through Step 6
Fine	100	_____	_____	_____	_____
Regular	400	_____	_____	_____	_____
Fast	800	_____	_____	_____	_____

ANALYSIS

1. Were the differences in contrast of the four images significant? Explain.

2. Based on your data, what conclusions can you draw about the effect of screen speed on image contrast?

3. Would you expect to see a difference in image contrast between screens of the same speed and phosphor type but matched with different film? Explain.

4. Would you expect to see a difference in contrast between screens of the same speed but of different phosphor types? Explain.

LABORATORY 29-3 THE EFFECT OF SUBJECT DENSITY AND CONTRAST ON IMAGE CONTRAST

PURPOSE

Demonstrate the effect of different subject densities and contrast on image contrast.

FOR FURTHER REVIEW

Refer to Chapter 29 in the accompanying textbook for further review of this topic.

MATERIALS

1. Energized radiographic unit

2. Automatic film processor

3. 8″ × 10″ radiographic cassettes with film

4. Shallow container (about 3″ to 4″ deep)

5. Ice cubes

6. 35 mm film canister

7. Super ball 1″ diameter size

8. Barium solution

SUGGESTED EXPOSURE FACTORS

100 RS, see procedure for mAs and kVp, 40″ SID, nongrid

PROCEDURES

Use the films produced for Laboratory 28-6, The Effect of Subject Density and Contrast on Density. If Laboratory 28-6 was not done previously, use the procedures section from that laboratory to produce the image for this laboratory.

RESULTS

1. Review the exposures on both images for image contrast.

ANALYSIS

1. What caused the different contrast ranges seen in image #1?

2. Why was the contrast reduced in the second exposure on image #1?

LABORATORY 29-3 (Continued)

3. Which exposure demonstrates the greatest contrast on image #2? Why?

4. Which exposure demonstrates the least contrast on image #2? Why?

5. Assuming the super ball is a solid tumor, which of the first three images demonstrates its contrast the best? Why?

LABORATORY 29-4 THE EFFECT OF EXPOSURE LATITUDE ON IMAGE CONTRAST

PURPOSE

Demonstrate how exposure latitude affects image contrast.

FOR FURTHER REVIEW

Refer to Chapter 29 in the accompanying textbook for further review of this topic.

MATERIALS

1. Energized radiographic unit

2. Automatic film processor

3. 10″ × 12″ radiographic cassettes with image receptor

4. Hand phantom

SUGGESTED EXPOSURE FACTORS

100 RS, see procedure for mAs and kVp, 40″ SID, nongrid

PROCEDURES

1. Mask a cassette in half crosswise and center it to the top of the radiographic table. Center the hand phantom to the unmasked portion of the cassette, label it exposure #1, collimate to the film size, and expose using 45 kVp and 20 mAs.

2. Repeat step 1, labeling it exposure 2, expose using 55 kVp and 20 mAs, and process the image receptor.

3. Repeat steps 1 and 2. Label the first half exposure #3 and expose using 73 kVp and 5 mAs. Label the second half exposure #4 and expose using 83 kVp and 5 mAs. Process the image receptor.

4. Repeat steps 1 and 2. Label the first half exposure #5 and expose using 96 kVp and 1 mAs. Label the second half exposure #6 and expose using 106 kVp and 1 mAs. Process the image receptor.

5. Place a CR cassette on top of the radiographic table and center the hand phantom to the center of the cassette. Center and collimate the central ray to the hand and expose using 45 kVp, 8mAs. Process the image using a hand algorithm and label the image #7.

6. Repeat step 5 using 55 kVp, 8mAs for image #8; 73 kVp, 2 mAs for image #9; 83 kVp, 2 mAs for image #10; 96 kVp, 1 mAs for image #11; and 106 kVp, 1 mAs for image #12.

RESULTS

1. Review the screen/film and digital images with respect to radiographic density and image contrast.

ANALYSIS

1. Is the background exposure similar on all three images?

LABORATORY 29-4 (Continued)

2. For both the screen/film and digital images, which image demonstrates the lowest contrast? What is the reason for this?

3. For both the screen/film and digital images, which image demonstrates the highest contrast? What is the reason for this?

4. For both the screen/film and digital images, which image demonstrates the greatest difference between the contrast of the two exposures? Explain.

5. For both the screen/film and digital images, which image demonstrates the least difference between the contrast of the two exposures? Explain.

6. Summarize the effect that kVp has on exposure latitude, using the laboratory results to support your statements.

7. Explain the practical clinical application that is supported by the results of this laboratory activity.

LABORATORY 29-5 THE EFFECT OF GRIDS ON IMAGE CONTRAST

PURPOSE

Demonstrate the effectiveness of radiographic grids in the improvement of image contrast.

FOR FURTHER REVIEW

Refer to Chapter 29 in the accompanying textbook for further review of this topic.

MATERIALS

1. Energized radiographic unit

2. Automatic film processor

3. Low- and high-ratio radiographic grids

4. Abdomen phantom

5. 14″ × 17″ radiographic cassettes with image receptors

6. Step wedge (penetrometer)

7. Densitometer

SUGGESTED EXPOSURE FACTORS

400 RS, 200 mA, 0.03 sec, 75 kVp, 40″ SID, nongrid

PROCEDURES

1. Center the abdomen phantom to the cassette on the tabletop. Place the step wedge beside the phantom on the cassette. Direct the central ray perpendicular and collimate to the edges of the cassette.

2. Using the suggested exposure factors, expose the image receptors, process, and label it #1.

3. Use a densitometer to measure the OD of steps 4, 5, and 6 on the penetrometer and record the readings. The OD of step 5 should be 1.2 ± 0.2. If not, adjust the mAs and reexpose.

4. Repeat the procedure using a low-ratio grid. Expose the image receptor using the appropriate grid conversion factor, process, and label it #2.

5. Repeat the procedure using a high ratio grid. Expose the image receptor using the appropriate grid conversion factor, process, and label it #3.

6. Calculate the image contrast of each image by subtracting the OD of step 6 from the OD of step 4.

LABORATORY 29-5 (Continued)

RESULTS

1. Review the three images in terms of their exposure and contrast.

	Step Wedge Optical Density			Contrast
	Step 4	Step 5	Step 6	Step 4 through Step 6
Image #1	_____	_____	_____	_____
Image #2	_____	_____	_____	_____
Image #3	_____	_____	_____	_____

ANALYSIS

1. Compare the radiographic densities and image contrast of images 1, 2, and 3. Which image(s) more closely approximate(s) a quality image? Why?

2. Where are the differences in image contrast of the three images significant? Explain.

3. Based on your data, what conclusions can you draw about the effect of grids and grid ratio on image contrast?

4. What factors or influences have contributed to the decrease or increase of image quality in each of the images?

5. Why is a radiographic grid important?

Name _____ Course _____ Date _____

LABORATORY 30-1 THE EFFECT OF DISTANCE ON RECORDED DETAIL

PURPOSE

Demonstrate the effects of object film distance and source image receptor distance on recorded detail.

FOR FURTHER REVIEW

Refer to Chapter 30 in the accompanying textbook for further review of this topic.

MATERIALS

1. Energized radiographic unit

2. 8″ × 10″ cassettes and image receptor

3. Dry bone parts

4. Radiolucent sponges

5. Lead masks

6. Resolution test pattern

7. Film processor

SUGGESTED EXPOSURE FACTORS

100 RS, 1.7 mAs, 55 kVp, 40″ SID, nongrid

PROCEDURES

1. Mask a cassette in half and place the test pattern and a dry bone on a 2″ radiolucent sponge on the unmasked portion of the cassette. Center the bone and test pattern to the unmasked half, label it exposure #1, collimate to the edges of the unmasked area, and expose it using 55 kVp, 3 mAs, and 40″ SID.

2. Readjust the mask to the other half of the cassette, center the bone and test pattern on top of an 8 sponge on the unmasked portion of the cassette, label it exposure #2, collimate to the unmasked area, and expose it using the same technical factors, and process the film.

3. Place a cassette on the floor, mask it in half and place the test pattern and dry bone on an 8 radiolucent sponge on the unmasked portion of the cassette. Center the bone and test pattern to the unmasked half, label it exposure #3, collimate it to the edges of the unmasked area, and expose it using 55 kVp and 60″ SID with the mAs adjusted according to the density maintenance formula (as derived from the inverse square law) to maintain the same density as the first film.

LABORATORY 30-1 (Continued)

RESULTS

1. Review all four images. Compare the recorded detail of both the bone and the test pattern images. Carefully determine the image of the smallest group where the line pairs can be distinctly defined (separated) and record the lines/mm of the group below.

<u>Smallest Group Resolved (lines/mm)</u>

40″ SID/2″ OID   _____

40″ SID/8″ OID   _____

60″ SID/8″ OID   _____

ANALYSIS

1. Is there an obvious loss of recorded detail between the first two exposures of the bone? Which image demonstrates the best recorded detail?

2. On exposures #1 and #2, is the recorded detail loss as great in the test pattern as with the bone? Explain the reasons for the difference, if any. Indicate the greatest number of lines/mm demonstrated on each exposure.

3. Describe the recorded detail of exposures #2 and #3. What is the greatest number of lines/mm that you can clearly see? What causes this difference? Explain.

4. Describe the effect of SID as it relates to image definition. Of what practical value is this knowledge to the radiographer?

LABORATORY 30-2 THE EFFECT OF FOCAL SPOT SIZE ON RECORDED DETAIL

PURPOSE

Demonstrate the effect of focal spot size on recorded detail.

FOR FURTHER REVIEW

Refer to Chapter 30 in the accompanying textbook for further review of this topic.

MATERIALS

1. Energized radiographic unit

2. Automatic film processor

3. 8″ × 10″ cassette and image receptor

4. Dry bones

5. Resolution test pattern

6. Radiolucent sponge

SUGGESTED EXPOSURE FACTORS

100 RS, 100 mA, 0.017 sec, 55 kVp, 40″ SID, nongrid

PROCEDURES

1. Ascertain that the exposure factors to be used can be obtained with both a small and large focal spot. If not, locate a radiographic unit capable of satisfying this requirement.

2. Mask the cassette in half, center a dry bone and the test pattern on a 2″ thick radiolucent sponge to the unmasked side, label it exposure #1, and then collimate and expose it using the small focal spot.

3. Repeat step 2 on the other half of the cassette, label exposure #2, expose it using the large focal spot, and process the film.

RESULTS

1. Review both images. Compare the recorded detail of both the bone and the test pattern images. Carefully determine the image of the smallest group where the line pairs can be distinctly defined and record the lp/mm as follows.

Smallest Group Resolved (lp/mm)

Small Focal Spot   _____

Large Focal Spot   _____

LABORATORY 30-2 (Continued)

ANALYSIS

1. Is there an obvious loss of recorded detail between the two images of the bone? Which image demonstrates the best detail?

2. Is there an obvious loss of recorded detail between the two resolution test patterns? Indicate the greatest number of lp/mm that you can see clearly defined in each of the images.

3. Is this loss as appreciable as that demonstrated in the images of the bones? Explain the reasons for your conclusion.

LABORATORY 30-3 THE EFFECT OF FILM/SCREEN COMBINATIONS ON RECORDED DETAIL

PURPOSE

Demonstrate the effect of different radiographic film/screen combinations on recorded detail.

FOR FURTHER REVIEW

Refer to Chapter 30 in the accompanying textbook for further review of this topic.

MATERIALS

1. Energized radiographic unit

2. Automatic film processor

3. Various speed cassettes with image receptors

4. Hand phantom

5. Resolution test pattern

6. Radiolucent sponge

SUGGESTED EXPOSURE FACTORS

See procedure.

PROCEDURES

1. Place the line pair test tool on a 2″ radiolucent sponge, position it next to the phantom hand, expose a film with each of the three different intensifying screens listed below using a 40″ SID and the suggested exposure factors, and process the films.

100 RS (fine)	54 kVp, 25 mA, 3/20 sec
400 RS (regular)	54 kVp, 25 mA, 1/20 sec
800 RS (fast)	54 kVp, 25 mA, 1/40 sec

RESULTS

1. Review all three images. Compare the recorded detail of both the hand and the test pattern images. Carefully determine the image of the smallest group where the line pairs can be distinctly defined (separated) and record the lines/mm of the group below.

Smallest Group Resolved (lines/mm)

100 RS	_____
400 RS	_____
800 RS	_____

LABORATORY 30-3 (Continued)

ANALYSIS

1. Is the difference in recorded detail displayed on the three images more noticeable with the hand images or the test pattern images. Why?

2. Which image exhibits the best recorded detail? Support your choice by describing the images.

3. Which image demonstrates the poorest recorded detail? Support your choice by describing the images.

4. List the factors associated with intensifying screens that have an impact on recorded detail and use these factors to explain the results you obtained.

5. What clinical trade-off is apparent when selecting a screen that produces better recorded detail?

LABORATORY 30-4 THE EFFECT OF MOTION ON RECORDED DETAIL

PURPOSE

Demonstrate the effect of object motion on recorded detail.

FOR FURTHER REVIEW

Refer to Chapter 30 in the accompanying textbook for further review of this topic.

MATERIALS

1. Energized radiographic unit

2. Automatic film processor

3. Nonscreen film holder with image receptor

4. Hand phantom

5. String

SUGGESTED EXPOSURE FACTORS

Direct exposure, 100 mA, 3.0 sec, 62 kVp, 40″ SID, nongrid

PROCEDURES

1. Mask a nonscreen film holder in half, center the hand phantom to the unmasked area, direct a perpendicular CR to the center of the hand, collimate to the unmasked section, and expose.

2. Remask to the other half and repeat step 1 with the hand in motion. Motion can be achieved by tying to the phantom a piece of string of sufficient length to reach the control booth and gently pulling the phantom during the exposure. (It is best to practice several times before making the exposure.) Then process the film.

RESULTS

1. Review both radiographic images. Consider the recorded detail of each image.

ANALYSIS

1. Is there a difference between the recorded detail of the two images? If a difference is noted, describe it.

2. Why does motion reduce recorded detail?

LABORATORY 30-4 (Continued)

3. List the two types of patient motion associated with imaging. Give two methods that could be used to control each type.

LABORATORY 31-1 THE EFFECT OF DISTANCE ON SIZE DISTORTION

PURPOSE

Demonstrate the effect of OID and SID on size distortion.

FOR FURTHER REVIEW

Refer to Chapter 31 in the accompanying textbook for further review of this topic.

MATERIALS

1. Energized radiographic unit
2. Automatic film processor
3. 10″ × 12″ cassette with image receptor
4. Small dry bone (vertebra preferred)
5. Metric ruler

SUGGESTED EXPOSURE FACTORS

100 RS, 100 mA, 0.017 sec, 55 kVp, 40″ SID, nongrid

PROCEDURES

OID Procedure

1. Mask a cassette in quarters, center a dry bone on a 2″ thick radiolucent sponge to the unmasked area, label exposure #1, collimate, and expose.

2. Repeat step 1 on an unmasked area, using another sponge to increase the OID to 4″, label exposure #2, and expose.

3. Repeat step 1 on an unmasked area, using another sponge to increase the OID to 8″, label exposure #3, and expose.

4. Repeat step 1 on an unmasked area, using another sponge to increase the OID to 12″, label exposure #4, expose, and process the film.

SID Procedure

1. Mask a cassette in quarters, center a dry bone on a 2″ thick radiolucent sponge to the unmasked area, change the SID to 20″, use the exposure maintenance formula (as derived from the inverse square law) to adjust the exposure factors, label exposure #1, collimate, and expose.

2. Repeat step 1 on an unmasked area, using 30″ SID, use the exposure maintenance formula to adjust the exposure factors, label exposure #2, and expose.

3. Repeat step 1 on an unmasked area, using 40″ SID, use the exposure maintenance formula to adjust the exposure factors, label exposure #2, and expose.

LABORATORY 31-1 (Continued)

4. Repeat step 1 on an unmasked area, using 60″ SID (this distance is best obtained by placing the cassette on the floor), use the exposure maintenance formula to adjust the exposure factors, label exposure #2, and expose.

RESULTS

1. Accurately record the length of the dry bone and the images from the various exposures.

2. Calculate and record the magnification factor and percentage of magnification for each image.

OID DATA FORM

DRY BONE (OBJECT) LENGTH (OL) = _____ mm   SID = _____

OID	Bone Image Length (IL) (mm)	Magnification Factor (m) $$\dfrac{SID}{SID - OID}$$	% Magnification (% M) $$\dfrac{IL - OL}{OL} \times 100$$
2″			
4″			
8″			
12″			

SID DATA FORM

DRY BONE (OBJECT) LENGTH (OL) = _____ mm   OID = _____

OID	mAs	Bone Image Length (IL) (mm)	Magnification Factor (m) $$\dfrac{SID}{SID - OID}$$	% Magnification (% M) $$\dfrac{IL - OL}{OL} \times 100$$
20″				
30″				
40″				
60″				

ANALYSIS

1. What happens to the recorded size of the image as the OID increases?

2. At what point does the loss of image detail become unacceptable? Explain.

3. What happens to the recorded size of the image as the SID increases?

4. At what point does the loss of image detail become unacceptable? Explain.

5. Describe the role of SID in producing size distortion and indicate how you would use this information to your advantage to produce an image with minimal size distortion.

6. Compare the results of the two Procedures. Which factor produces the greatest influence on size distortion? Support your answer.

7. Do the magnification factor and percentages compare favorably? Explain.

8. What effect does size distortion have on recorded detail?

Name _____ Course _____ Date _____

LABORATORY 31-2 THE EFFECT OF ALIGNMENT AND ANGULATION ON SHAPE DISTORTION

PURPOSE

Demonstrate the effect of part/image receptor alignment, central ray/part/image receptor alignment and central ray direction on shape distortion.

FOR FURTHER REVIEW

Refer to Chapter 31 in the accompanying textbook for further review of this topic.

MATERIALS

1. Energized radiographic unit

2. Automatic film processor

3. 10″ × 12″ cassette with image receptor

4. Dry bone

5. Metric ruler

SUGGESTED EXPOSURE FACTORS

100 RS, 100 mA, 0.017 sec, 55 kVp, 40″ SID, nongrid

PROCEDURES

Part/Image Receptor Alignment

1. Position a 10″ × 12″ cassette lengthwise on the tabletop so the ID blocker is down, mask the cassette in thirds lengthwise, tape the dry bone on a 4″ sponge so that the long axis of the bone is parallel to the tube axis, center the bone to an unmasked area, direct the central ray to the center of the bone with a 40″ SID, label exposure #1, and expose.

2. Repeat step 1 on an unexposed area, center the bone to the area, direct the central ray to the center of the bone with a 40″ SID, raise the right (cathode) end of the sponge so the bone forms a 30° angle with the film plane, label exposure #2, and expose.

3. Repeat step 1 on an unexposed area, center the bone to the area, direct the central ray to the center of the bone with a 40″ SID, raise the left (anode) end of the sponge so the bone forms a 30° angle with the film plane, label exposure #3, expose, and process the receptor.

CR/Part/Image Receptor Alignment

1. Position a 10″ × 12″ cassette lengthwise on the tabletop so the ID blocker is down, mask the cassette in thirds lengthwise, tape the dry bone on a 4″ sponge so that the long axis of the bone is parallel to the tube axis, center the bone to an unmasked area, direct the central ray to the center of the bone with a 40″ SID, label exposure #4, and expose.

2. Repeat step 1 on an unmasked area, center the bone to the area, direct the central ray to the left (toward the anode) along the longitudinal axis of the bone until it is 6″ off-center, open the collimator to include the entire bone, label exposure #5, and expose.

LABORATORY 31–2 (Continued)

3. Repeat step 1 on an unmasked area, center the bone to the area, direct the central ray to the right (toward the cathode) along the longitudinal axis of the bone until it is 6″ off-center, open the collimator to include the entire bone, label exposure #6, expose, and process the receptor.

Central Ray Direction

1. Position a 10″ × 12″ cassette lengthwise on the tabletop so the ID blocker is down, mask the cassette in thirds lengthwise, tape the dry bone on a 4″ sponge so that the long axis of the bone is parallel to the tube axis, center the bone to an unmasked area, direct the central ray to the center of the bone with a 40″ SID, label exposure #7, and expose.

2. Repeat step 1 on an unmasked area, center the bone to the area, direct the central ray to the left (toward the anode) along the longitudinal axis of the bone until it is 6″ off-center, angle back 25° to the original centering point, reduce the SID to 40″, label exposure #8, and expose.

3. Repeat step 2 on an unmasked area, direct the central ray to the right (toward the cathode) along the longitudinal axis of the bone until it is 6″ off-center, angle back 25° to the original centering point, reduce the SID to 40″, label exposure #9, expose, and process the receptor.

RESULTS

1. Accurately measure the length of the dry bone and the images of the bone on the image receptor and record them in mm.

Dry Bone Length _____ mm   Bone Image Length (mm)

Part/IR Alignment	Image 1	Image 2	Image 3
	_____	_____	_____
Central Ray/Part/IR Alignment	Image 4	Image 5	Image 6
	_____	_____	_____
Central Ray Direction	Image 7	Image 8	Image 9
	_____	_____	_____

ANALYSIS

Part/IR Alignment

1. Compare the differences in anatomical appearance between the recorded images in which portions are elongated/foreshortened. Compare image 1 to 2, 1 to 3, and 2 to 3.

2. Can shape distortion caused by improper part/image receptor relationship also contribute to size distortion? Explain.

3. To minimize shape distortion, indicate the most ideal relationship between the structures of interest and the film plane.

Central Ray/Part/Image Receptor Alignment

4. Compare the differences in anatomical appearance between the recorded images in which portions are elongated/foreshortened. Compare image 4 to 5, 4 to 6, and 5 to 6.

5. Can shape distortion caused by improper central ray/part/IR alignment also contribute to size distortion? Explain.

6. Describe the significance of off-centering of the central ray on the visualization of joint spaces or nondisplaced fractures.

Central Ray Direction

7. Compare the differences in anatomical appearance between the recorded images in which portions are elongated/foreshortened. Compare image 7 to 8, 7 to 9, and 8 to 9.

8. Can shape distortion caused by improper central ray direction through the part also contribute to size distortion? Explain.

LABORATORY 31-2 (Continued)

9. Would it be more appropriate to direct the central ray perpendicular to the image receptor or to the structure of interest? Explain your answer and provide some practical examples that support your position.

10. Compare the shape distortion produced in the three different scenarios. Of the three causes of shape distortion identified, which produces the most obvious misrepresentation of the structure? Support your answer with examples.

11. Name three examinations/projections in which shape distortion is used to best advantage and describe how this is accomplished.

LABORATORY 32-1 IMAGE CRITIQUE: ASSESSING DENSITY, CONTRAST, RECORDED DETAIL, AND DISTORTION

PURPOSE

Critique images effectively.

FOR FURTHER REVIEW

Refer to Chapter 32 in the accompanying textbook for further review of this topic.

MATERIALS

1. A repeated image

PROCEDURES

1. Use the procedures described in Chapter 32 of the textbook to critique the repeated images, using the following form.

ANALYSIS

IMAGE CRITIQUE FORM

I.   CLASSIFY THE RADIOGRAPHIC IMAGE AS:
☐ **WITHIN ACCEPTANCE LIMITS**
    ☐ Optimal diagnostic information (critique is complete)
<u>(all checkmarks below this line require completion of section II and III)</u>
    ☐ Suboptimal diagnostic information
☐ **OUTSIDE ACCEPTANCE LIMITS**

II. DETERMINE THE CAUSE OF THE PROBLEM AS:
☐   **A:**   **Technical Factors**
    ☐ Photographic problem with visibility of detail
        ☐ Density
            ☐ mAs_____
            ☐ Influencing factor (specify) _____
        ☐ Contrast
            ☐ kVp _____
            ☐ Influencing factor (specify) _____
    ☐ Geometric problem with detail
        ☐ Recorded detail
            ☐ Geometry (specify) _____
            ☐ Image Receptor _____
            ☐ Motion _____
        ☐ Distortion
            ☐ Size (Magnification) (specify)_____
            ☐ Shape (Part/Image Receptor /Tube Alignment) (specify) _____
☐   **B:**   **Procedural Factors**
    ☐ Patient Positioning
        ☐ Tube Alignment _____
        ☐ Part Alignment _____
        ☐ Image Receptor Alignment _____
    ☐ Patient Preparation (specify) _____
☐   **C:**   **Equipment Malfunction**
    ☐ Processing Equipment (specify) _____
    ☐ Radiographic/Fluoroscopic Equipment (specify) _____

III. RECOMMENDED CORRECTIVE ACTION For each cause specified above:
_____
_____
_____
_____

LABORATORY 33-1 PROCESSOR SENSITOMETRIC MONITORING CHARTS

PURPOSE

Monitor an automatic film processor sensitometrically.

FOR FURTHER REVIEW

Refer to Chapter 33 in the accompanying textbook for further review of this topic.

MATERIALS

1. Automatic film processor
2. Sensitometer
3. Densitometer
4. Radiographic control film
5. Photographic thermometer

PROCEDURES

1. A quantity (box) of radiographic film that is normally used in the processor being monitored should be set aside to be used as control film. Use this film when making the sensitometric control strips.

2. Using a sheet of film from the control box, expose the film in the sensitometer. Follow the sensitometer's instruction manual for the correct procedure.

3. Process the sensitometric film. If the monitoring activity is going to be over a period of time, then the test film should be processed in a like fashion each time (i.e., film orientation, feed tray position, etc.).

4. Measure the developer temperature, using a photographic thermometer each time a control film is processed. Record the temperature reading in the appropriate section of the processor monitoring record.

5. Use the densitometer to measure and record the step numbers and their optical densities on the sensitometric control strip for the following monitoring parameters:

Contrast Index

The OD of the step closest to but not less than 2.20 OD minus the OD of the step closest to but not greater than 0.45 OD.

Speed Index

Step closest to 1.20 OD.

Base + Fog Index

Unexposed portion of test film or first step.

LABORATORY 33–1 (Continued)

6. These Procedures will be used to measure these parameters, assuming that the processor is currently operating normally. The parameters measured previously will be considered the normal value for this activity. Record these measurements (step numbers and densities) in the appropriate section of the processor monitoring record.

7. Monitor a film processor over a period of 2 to 4 weeks. The processor should be tested at least once a day at a time during its active use, using freshly sensitized sensitometric control strips. Record the developer temperature and the OD of each of the parameters on the processor monitoring record each time a sensitometric control strip is processed.

Acceptance Criteria

Each parameter should test within control limits for the processor to be considered operating normally and consistently. The control limits are:

Contrast Index:	plus or minus 0.10 OD
Speed Index:	plus or minus 0.10 OD
Base + Fog Index:	plus or minus 0.05 OD
Developer Temp:	plus or minus 1° F or 0.5° C

RESULTS

See page 178.

ANALYSIS

1. If this activity required you to monitor a processor over a period of time, did any of the parameters fall outside of the control limits? What was the cause? How was the situation corrected?

2. Why is it recommended that freshly sensitized sensitometric control strips be used rather than presensitizing a quantity of strips and using them throughout the monitoring procedure?

3. What effect would you predict for the speed, contrast, and base + fog indexes if the following occurred?

   a. Five hundred 14″ × 17″ films are run through the processor instead of 500 intermixed sized films.

b. The incoming water supply to the processor was 95° F when it should be 90° F.

c. A cracked safelight filter was found.

4. Discuss the importance of processor maintenance and its impact on processor quality control.

LABORATORY 33-1 (Continued)

MONTH _____ YEAR _____
PROCESSOR MODEL NO. _____
LOCATION _____
RECORDED BY _____

| | 1 | 3 | 5 | 7 | 9 | 11 | 13 | 15 | 17 | 19 | 21 | 23 | 25 | 27 | 29 | 31 |

SPEED STEP NO. _____

+0.20 _____
+0.15 _____
+0.10 _____
+0.05 _____
D
–0.05 _____
–0.10 _____
–0.15 _____
–0.20 _____

CONTRAST
STEP _____ –STEP _____

+0.20 _____
+0.15 _____
+0.10 _____
+0.05 _____
D
–0.05 _____
–0.10 _____
–0.15 _____
–0.20 _____

GROSS FOG STEP _____

+0.10 _____
+0.05 _____
D
–0.05 _____
–0.10 _____

DEVELOPER STANDARD TEMP. _____ °

+10° _____
+5° _____
–5° _____
–10° _____

LABORATORY 33-2 ESTIMATING FOCAL SPOT SIZE

PURPOSE

Evaluate focal spot size using a star x-ray test pattern.

FOR FURTHER REVIEW

Refer to Chapter 33 in the accompanying textbook for further review of this topic.

MATERIALS

1. Energized radiographic unit

2. Automatic film processor

3. 1.5 or 2 degree star x-ray test pattern

4. 10″ × 12″ nonscreen film holder with screen film

5. Small metric ruler

SUGGESTED EXPOSURE FACTORS

Screen film with direct exposure, 20 mAs, 75 kVp, 24″ SID, nongrid

PROCEDURES

1. Locate the tube identification plate attached to the x-ray tube housing of the unit being tested. Record the nominal (manufacturer's specification) focal spot sizes that are indicated on the plate for the x-ray tube. They often appear as simply single decimal numbers (for example, 0.6 to 2.0 to indicate 0.6 mm and 2.0 mm focal spots).

2. Activate the collimator localizer light of the x-ray tube being evaluated, place the star test pattern in contact with the faceplate of the collimator so it is centered to the center, and rotate the star so one set of lead lines is parallel with the long axis of the tube and the other set is perpendicular. Tape the test pattern to the collimator faceplate in this position.

3. Center the loaded film holder lengthwise on the radiographic table, mask it in half crosswise, adjust the central ray perpendicular to the center of the unmasked area, label the anode and cathode sides of the film holder, use a 24″ SID, collimate to the unmasked portion of the film holder, select the large focal spot, and expose.

4. Readjust the mask, repeat step 2 using the small focal spot, expose, and process the film. An OD of 1.2 to 1.5 should be obtained if possible.

5. Determine the magnification (M) factor by dividing the diameter of the radiographic image of the star test pattern by the true diameter of the star test pattern.

6. Determine the point at which failure of resolution occurs. By viewing the image starting at the outer margin of the star pattern, move inward to the first area of blurring and mark this point. Mark the point where failure of resolution occurs on all four sides. Measure the distance in millimeters between the two marks along the anode cathode axis (D1) to determine the width of the focal spot. Measure the distance in millimeters between the two marks perpendicular to the anode cathode axis (D2) to determine the length of the focal spot.

7. Calculate the equivalent focal spot size (F_{mm}) according to the following formula:

$$F_{mm} = [N \div 57.3] \times [D \div (M - 1)]$$

where:

N = the angle of the star pattern used for the evaluation, that is, 1.5 or 2

D = distance between failure of resolution marks in mm

M = magnification factor

F_{mm} = equivalent focal spot size in mm

RESULTS

	Small Focal Spot	Large Focal Spot
Nominal Size	_____	_____
Equivalent Size	_____	_____

ANALYSIS

1. What are the measured equivalent sizes of the large and small focal spots?

2. How do these figures compare to the nominal (manufacturer specified) focal spot size for the tube evaluated? If they are larger, do they meet the acceptable tolerance limits specified by NEMA (see textbook Chapter 6)? Explain.

3. Describe another method that can be used to evaluate focal spot size.

4. Describe the differences between effective, equivalent, and actual focal spot size.

LABORATORY 33-3 EVALUATING COLLIMATOR, CENTRAL RAY, AND BUCKY TRAY ALIGNMENT

PURPOSE

Evaluate the alignment of the light field and central ray to the x-ray beam and Bucky tray as well as the accuracy of the automatic collimation system.

FOR FURTHER REVIEW

Refer to Chapter 33 in the accompanying textbook for further review of this topic.

MATERIALS

1. Energized radiographic unit equipped with PBL

2. Automatic film processor

3. Various size radiographic cassettes with image receptors

4. One sheet of scrap film for each cassette size

5. Four paper clips

6. Collimator alignment template or nine pennies

7. X-ray beam perpendicularity test tool

SUGGESTED EXPOSURE FACTORS

400 RS, 25 mA, 0.05 sec, 55 kVp, 40″ SID, nongrid

PROCEDURES

Light Field X-ray Beam Alignment and Perpendicularity

1. Center the alignment template on the cassette and place it on the tabletop.

2. Center the light field to the cross centering mark on the template using 40″ SID.

3. Switch the PBL to manual mode and adjust the collimator light field to the field marks on the template.

4. If the light field is centered to the template, and one or more of the edges of the light field are not on the corresponding field marks, place straightened paper clips on the edges of the light field to mark the location.

5. Place the perpendicularity test tool on the template, making sure it is exactly centered to the template and to the center of the light field.

6. Place ID markers on the tabletop in the quadrant of the light field that represents the right shoulder of a supine patient for orientation purposes in the event misalignment is noted and expose the receptor.

7. Open the collimator to cover the entire receptor, expose a second time using half the mAs (this will be a double exposure), and process the receptor.

8. Evaluate the image for x-ray beam to light field alignment.

Acceptance Limits

1. Federal guidelines for certified equipment allow ± 2 percent of the SID for x-ray beam to light field alignment. The edges of the radiation field should be within ± 1 cm of the template markers indicating the location of the light field edges.

2. The image of the BBs in the perpendicularity test tool should appear within 5 mm of one another.

Nine-Penny Test for Beam Alignment

1. Center a 10″ × 12″ cassette on the x-ray tabletop with its long dimension parallel to the long dimension of the table.

2. Center the light field to the center of the cassette at a 40″ SID.

3. Manually collimate the x-ray beam to a 6″ × 8″ field size.

4. Position two pennies in the center of each margin of the light field so that one entire penny is inside the light field and one is outside the light field. Place the ninth penny in the quadrant of the light field that represents the right shoulder of a supine patient as an orientation marker.

5. Place lead markers well inside the light field on the cassette to identify the room number and date and expose the film at about 55 kVp and 1.25 mAs.

6. Open the collimator and adjust the light field size to the cassette and expose the cassette again using 55 kVp and 0.5 mAs (this will be a double exposure), and process the receptor.

7. Evaluate the accuracy of the x-ray field.

Acceptance Limits

Federal guidelines for certified equipment allow ± 2 percent of the SID for the x-ray to light field alignment. For a 100 cm (40″) SID, ± 2 cm (one penny) is acceptable. The x-ray to light field should be well within this guideline. Alignment to ± 1 cm (± 0.5 penny) can reasonably be achieved.

Field Size versus Cassette Size for Automatic Collimation (PBL) Systems

1. Set the x-ray tube at the usual source-to-image receptor distance used for Bucky radiographs.

2. Set the PBL selector to the automatic mode.

3. Insert each size of cassette commonly used in the Bucky tray lengthwise and then transversely. Visually check that the changes in the light field size occur with the changes in cassette size and that the size of the light field is appropriate by comparing the light field size to the film size using scrap film sheets.

Acceptance Limits

Federal guidelines for certified equipment allow ± 3 percent of the SID for PBL misalignment; however, a ± 1 cm is reasonably achievable.

LABORATORY 33-3 (Continued)

X-ray Field and Bucky Alignment

1. Set the x-ray tube to the transverse center position.

2. Place straightened paper clips on the x-ray tabletop along the crosshairs of the collimator light field.

3. Insert a 10″ × 12″ cassette lengthwise in the Bucky tray. Collimate the beam to an 8″ × 10″ size with the long dimension parallel to the x-ray tabletop.

4. Place ID markers on the tabletop in the quadrant of the light field that represents the right shoulder of a supine patient for orientation purposes in the event misalignment is noted and expose using about 50 kVp and 5 mAs.

5. Measure the distance from the center of the radiographic image as indicated by the crossed paper clips to the edges of the exposed portion of the image and to the edges of the receptor.

Acceptance Limits

The exposed portion of the image should be centered to the film within ± 1 cm in both length and width. The center indicated by the images of the crossed paper clips should actually be centered to the exposed portion of the image to within ± 1 cm.

RESULTS

1. Evaluate all the test images against the acceptance criteria.

ANALYSIS

1. Was the radiation light field alignment within acceptable limits? Explain. Discuss the clinical implications of a misaligned radiation beam and light field.

2. Was the radiation beam centering and perpendicularity within acceptable limits? Explain. Discuss the clinical implications of misalignment of the center of the beam and a beam that is not perpendicular.

3. Was the PBL test within acceptable limits? If not, explain the unacceptable elements. Discuss the clinical implications of an improperly operating PBL device.

4. Was the Bucky tray beam center alignment within acceptable limits? Explain. Discuss the clinical implications of an improperly aligned Bucky tray.

5. List at least four causes of centering and radiation to light field misalignment.

LABORATORY 33-4 EVALUATING DISTANCE, CENTERING, AND ANGULATOR ACCURACY

PURPOSE

Evaluate the accuracy of an SID indicator, centering detent, and angulation indicator.

FOR FURTHER REVIEW

Refer to Chapter 33 in the accompanying textbook for further review of this topic.

MATERIALS

1. Energized radiographic unit

2. Automatic film processor

3. 8″ × 10″ cassette with image receptor

4. Quarter or other coin

5. Ring stand

6. Scrap film

7. Small ruler

8. Skull angulator or protractor

9. Small bubble level

SUGGESTED EXPOSURE FACTORS

400 RS, 100 mA, 0.0083 sec, 60 kVp, 40″ SID, 8:1 Bucky grid

PROCEDURES

SID Indicator Accuracy

1. Set up the ring stand on the tabletop 20 above the Bucky tray and center it on the table. Cut a 4″ × 4″ section from a scrap film and place it on the ring support. Center a quarter on the film, use the tube's SID indicator to position the tube 40 above the Bucky tray, center the central tray to the quarter and collimate appropriately. Place an 8″ × 10″ cassette in the Bucky tray and center it to the central ray, expose, and process.

2. Use a metric ruler to determine the diameter of the quarter (object size). Measure the diameter of the image of the quarter on the test film (image size). Calculate the SID using the following equation:

$$SID = \frac{Image\ size \times OID}{Image\ size - object\ size}$$

Tube Centering Detent Accuracy

1. Place the x-ray tube at the center detent position and visually inspect the tube housing from the end and front of the table to make sure it is not angled (a bubble level can be used for more accuracy). Turn on the light localizer and note the position of the crosshairs on the tabletop. The longitudinal crosshair should be aligned to the midline of the table.

Angulation Indicator Accuracy

1. Position the tube head so that the angulation indicator reads 0 degrees. Place the bubble level on top of the tube housing and determine if the bubble indicates a level tube position. Angle the tube in both directions and watch the indicator to see if it is accurate. A protractor or skull angulator can be used to verify the correct angle.

RESULTS

SID Indicator Accuracy

Indicated SID _____

Calculated SID _____

Angulation Indicator Accuracy

Angulation indicator reading
with tube head leveled _____

Tube Centering Detent Accuracy

Distance between crosshair
and table center line _____

ANALYSIS

1. What is the calculated SID?

2. The SID indicator should be within ± 2 percent of the calculated SID to be considered accurate. What is the percentage difference between the indicated SID and the calculated SID? Does the SID indicator pass the accuracy test?

3. Did the light localizer crosshair align with the midline of the table with the tube in the detent position? If not, by how much was it off?

4. Assume that the table did not have a center line. Describe a way that could be used to determine the accuracy of the detent mechanism.

5. Did the angulation indicator read 0 degrees with the tube head in a level position? If not, by how much was it off?

6. Describe at least one adverse effect that could result from each of the three parameters if they tested as being inaccurate.

LABORATORY 33-5 EVALUATING KILOVOLTAGE ACCURACY

PURPOSE

Evaluate the accuracy of kVp production.

FOR FURTHER REVIEW

Refer to Chapter 33 in the accompanying textbook for further review of this topic.

MATERIALS

1. Energized radiographic unit

2. Automatic film processor

3. Digital kVp meter or kVp test cassette (with current calibration curve)

4. Densitometer (required with kVp test cassette)

SUGGESTED EXPOSURE FACTORS

See procedure.

PROCEDURES

Digital kVp Meter

1. The kVp settings evaluated should represent common kVp and mAs settings. Evaluate 60, 70, 80, 90, and 100 kVp at two different mA stations. If the generator is used for fluoroscopy, evaluate 120 instead of 60 kVp.

2. Set the meter for radiographic testing and for three-phase or single-phase depending on the type of generator. Most meters should be warmed up by an exposure of about 100 mAs and 100 kVp.

3. Position the meter on the table so the LCD readout is visible from the control booth, the detector is centered to the x-ray beam at 40 source to detector distance, and collimate to approximately 6″ × 6″.

4. Set the desired kVp, use 100 ms or longer for three-phase generators and 200 ms or longer for single-phase generators (shorter exposure times [down to 50 ms] can be used without significant loss of accuracy), and expose.

5. Record the results. If no indication of sufficient intensity for a measurement occurs, decrease the source to detector distance or increase the mA. Do not change the kVp or time.

6. Repeat steps 3 through 5 for the remaining test exposures.

kVp Test Cassette

1. Follow the manufacturer's directions for specific information such as film type to be used with the test cassette, recommended SID, recommended mAs, and so on.

LABORATORY 33–5 (Continued)

2. Load the test cassette and place it on the tabletop so the long axis of the cassette is parallel to the anode-cathode axis of the x-ray tube. Center and collimate the x-ray beam to the cassette using the manufacturer's recommendation or a 36″ source-to-tabletop distance.

3. Set the generator to the mA station that will be used for all the kVp stations and identify the cassette with lead markers.

4. Mask the cassette in quarters and expose different areas of the cassette at 60, 80, 100, and 120 kVp. Adjust the time (not the mA) for each exposure so that an OD of 0.5 to 1.5 is produced for each exposure and process the film.

Approximate mAs techniques using 400 RS film and 36″ SID.

kVp	mAs	
	1 Phase	3 Phase
60	500	400
80	75	40
100	15	10
120	12	8

RESULTS
Digital kVp Meter

1. Record the kVp meter readings below.

Tested kVp	mA	Measured kVp
_____	_____	_____
_____	_____	_____
_____	_____	_____
_____	_____	_____
_____	_____	_____

2. The kVp on a properly calibrated generator should be maintained within ± 2 kVp. A variation of ± 5 kVp or more should be corrected by a service engineer.

kVp Test Cassette

1. Each kVp region on the image includes two columns of dots. Use a densitometer to measure the densities and record them on the data form. (The film must be repeated if the measured densities are not between OD 0.5 to 1.5.)

2. Locate the dot in the left (attenuation dot) column that most closely matches the densities in the right (reference dot) column.

LABORATORY 33-5 (Continued)

3. Unless an exact match is found, interpolate between the steps to determine the appropriate match dot number. For example:

	Attenuation Density	Reference Density
Step 5	1.10	1.05
Step 6	1.03	1.05

$$\text{Match Step} = 5 + \frac{1.10 - 1.05}{1.10 - 1.03} = 5 + \frac{0.05}{0.07} = 5.7$$

4. If the reference dots are not uniform in the area of the density match, determine the average density for the reference dots close to where the match occurs and use this average density for matching purposes.

5. After the match step has been determined for each of the kVp regions (steps 2 and 3), refer to the cassette's calibration curves to determine the kVp. Every test cassette is matched to its own calibration curve. The serial number of the cassette must match the number on the calibration curves. There is a separate chart for each kVp region and there is a separate curve on each chart for single- and three-phase generators.

6. Record the results below.

Tested kVp	Match Dot	Measured kVp
_____	_____	_____
_____	_____	_____
_____	_____	_____
_____	_____	_____
_____	_____	_____

7. The kVp on a properly calibrated generator should be maintained to within ± 2 kVp. A variation of ± 5 kVp or more should be corrected by a service engineer.

ANALYSIS

1. Were all the kVp settings tested within acceptable limits? If not, which ones were not and by how much?

2. Why is kVp considered such an important technical factor? Why must it be closely monitored?

3. What is the reason for aligning the long axis of the test cassette with the long axis of the x-ray tube?

4. Why do single- and three-phase generators require separate calibration curves to determine the kVp for this test?

5. If a problem with kVp calibration is suspected, why would viewing the output waveform be helpful?

6. What are two possible causes of kVp variations?

LABORATORY 33-6 EVALUATING TIMER ACCURACY

PURPOSE

Evaluate the accuracy of an exposure timer.

FOR FURTHER REVIEW

Refer to Chapter 33 in the accompanying textbook for further review of this topic.

MATERIALS

1. Energized radiographic unit

2. Automatic film processor

3. Motorized synchronous top, or digital exposure timer

4. 8″ × 10″ radiographic cassettes with image receptor

5. Timer protractor template or ordinary protractor

SUGGESTED EXPOSURE FACTORS

100 RS, 5 mAs, 75 kVp, 40″ SID, nongrid

Motorized Synchronous Top (for All Types of Generators)

1. The four exposures must be made using a constant mAs with varying mA and time. Typical values might be 0.2 sec @ 25 mA, 0.1 sec @ 50 mA, 0.05 sec @ 100 mA, and 0.03 sec @ 150 mA. Use mA stations that are commonly used with the generator.

2. Plug the timing tool in, mask the cassette in half and collimate. Center the top to the unmasked area, use 40″ SID, mark it #1, start the top spinning, and make the first exposure.

3. Change the mask and repeat step 2 for the remaining areas. Mark each appropriately, use different exposure factors for each, and process the film. Exposures #3 and 4 should be made with a second cassette.

4. Use the timer protractor template provided by the manufacturer to measure the angles of the darkened arcs, determine the time, and record it.

5. If the manufacturer's protractor template is not available, measure the angle of exposed arc using an ordinary protractor and use the following formula:

$$\frac{\text{Measured Angle}}{360° \times \text{RPS}} = \text{Exposure Time}$$

where: RPS is the revolutions per second at which the motor operates. For example, a 36° arc with a 1 RPS synchronous motor would be calculated as:

$$\frac{36°}{360° \times 1} = 0.1 \text{ second}$$

LABORATORY 33-6 (Continued)

Acceptance Criteria

For three-phase generators, exposure time error should be limited to ± 5 percent or ± 2 msec, whichever is larger.

Digital X-ray Exposure Timer (for All Types of Generators)

1. Turn the timer on. Select the appropriate measurement mode (Pulse—single phase, Time in sec, or Time in msec). Use the Time in sec mode for measuring times greater than 1/2 sec and the Time in msec for times less than 1/2 sec. Pulse mode will indicate the number of pulses delivered from a single-phase generator.

2. Position the meter level on the table so the LCD readout is visible from the control booth. The detector (indicated on the surface of the meter) is centered to the x-ray beam at a 40° source-to-detector distance. Collimate to the area of the detector.

3. Set the kVp at 80 and mA at 200. Select an exposure time to be tested and make an exposure.

4. Record the results. If meter displays obviously high or low values, notify your instructor.

5. Repeat steps 3 through 5 for three different exposure time settings for the remaining test exposures.

Acceptance Criteria

Use the same criteria previously given.

RESULTS

Motorized Synchronous Top

Time Station Tested	Measured Angle	Measured Exposure Time
_____	_____	_____
_____	_____	_____
_____	_____	_____
_____	_____	_____

Digital Exposure Timer

Time Station Tested	Measured Exposure Time
_____	_____
_____	_____
_____	_____
_____	_____

ANALYSIS

1. Were all the time stations evaluated within acceptable limits? If not, which ones were not and by how much?

2. What aspects of image quality are directly affected by exposure time?

3. An image of a motorized synchronous top demonstrates a measured arc of 90° when testing particular three-phase generators.

LABORATORY 33-7 EVALUATING EXPOSURE REPRODUCIBILITY, mA LINEARITY, AND mR/mAs

PURPOSE

Evaluate the reproducibility and linearity of a generator for commonly used exposure settings.

FOR FURTHER REVIEW

Refer to Chapter 33 in the accompanying textbook for further review of this topic.

MATERIALS

1. Energized radiographic unit

2. Digital dosimeter

SUGGESTED EXPOSURE FACTORS

Choose an mAs that will produce dosimeter readings in the range of 200 to 500 mR at 80 kVp.

PROCEDURES

1. Turn on the digital dosimeter, select the dose mode, and follow the manufacturer's instructions for the unit's operation.

2. Place the dosimeter detector (ionization chamber) on the radiographic table and using a 40″ source-to-detector distance, center and collimate the beam to the detector.

3. On the generator control panel, select 80 kVp, 100 mA, and an exposure time that will result in a dosimeter reading between 200 and 500 mR. Readjust the exposure time if necessary until the reading is within this range and record the values.

4. Randomly change the technical factor settings and then go back to the desired setting. Make three exposures and record the readings on the data form as X_1, X_2, and X_3, respectively.

5. Repeat steps 3 and 4, but use the next larger mA station (i.e., 200 mA).

6. Repeat steps 3 and 4, but use the next larger mA station (i.e., 300 mA).

7. Repeat steps 3 and 4, but use the next larger mA station (i.e., 400 mA).

8. In order to properly analyze the results of this test, certain simple calculations must be made and the results compared to the acceptance criteria.

   a. Calculate the average of the three exposure measurements made at each kVp, mA, and time combination and record on the data form.

$$\text{Average } X = (X_1 + X_2 + X_3)/3$$

b. Calculate the average exposure (Avg.) per indicated mAs for each mA and time station tested as:

$$\text{Avg. mR/mAs} = \text{Avg. X}/(\text{mA} \times \text{s})$$

where: Average X is the average value of the recorded exposures at each mA-time station combination and mA and s are the values of the stations selected. Record the calculated Avg. mR/mAs values on the data form.

c. For reproducibility calculate and record on the data form the ratios $X_1/\text{Avg. X}$, $X_2/\text{Avg. X}$, and $X_3/\text{Avg. X}$ for each kVp, mA, and time combination.

Acceptance Criteria

For any specific combination of selected technique factors, the exposures shall provide reproducible exposure to 0.05 or less. Thus, at a given kVp, mA, and time combination, the individual exposure measurements shall fall within 65 percent of the averages. This is indicated by $X_n/\text{Avg. X}$ ratios between 0.95 and 1.05.

d. For linearity, use the calculated mR/mAs values to determine the linearity across all the mA stations selected at 80 kVp.

$$\text{Linearity} = [(\text{Avg. mR/mAs})_{max} - (\text{Avg. mR/mAs})_{min}]/[(\text{Avg. mR/mAs})_{max} + (\text{Avg. mR/mAs})_{min}]$$

where: $(\text{Avg. mR/mAs})_{max}$ and $(\text{Avg. mR/mAs})_{min}$ are the maximum and minimum values of the calculated mR/mAs as recorded on the data form.

Acceptance Criteria

Essentially, linearity means that the ratio of exposure to total charge in mR/mAs is constant over the entire range of mAs values. The average mR/mAs obtained at any tube current settings (mA) shall not differ by more than 0.10. Linearity should be maintained to $\pm$ 10 percent over the entire working range of the generator regardless of the number of mA stations at a fixed kVp.

9. Generator output is determined by taking the average of the four mR/mAs values. Average output produced by diagnostic x-ray equipment with a total filtration of 2.5 mm Al measured at 80 kVp with a 40″ source-to-detector should be 5.0 mR/mAs for single phase and 8.0 mR/mAs for three phase.

Acceptance Criteria

The tested generator should agree with the average values to within $\pm$ 30 percent, assuming other tests indicate proper performance, that is, kVp, SID accuracy, HVL, and so forth.

RESULTS

1. Document the results of the test and calculations in the appropriate sections of the data form.

DATA FORM

mA							
Time							
mAs							
X_1							
X_2							
X_3							
Avg. X							
X_1/Avg. X							
X_2/Avg. X							
X_3/Avg. X							
Avg. mR/mAs							

ANALYSIS

1. Did the test results meet the acceptance criteria for reproducibility of the mA, linearity across mA stations, and output? If not, indicate which tests failed and support your conclusions.

2. Briefly discuss the importance of the reproducibility and linearity tests.

3. What might be a cause for reproducibility being unacceptable? Linearity?

4. Describe the benefits that can be derived from knowing the exposure output of the generators in a x-ray department. Why is exposure output expressed in mR/mAs?

LABORATORY 33-8 RADIOGRAPHIC CASSETTE QUALITY CONTROL

PURPOSE

Inspect and clean cassette screens and evaluate film/screen contact.

FOR FURTHER REVIEW

Refer to Chapter 33 in the accompanying textbook for further review of this topic.

MATERIALS

1. Energized radiographic unit

2. Automatic film processor

3. Cassettes

4. Screen cleaner solution

5. Gauze sponge pads

6. Wire mesh test pattern

7. Adhesive tape

SUGGESTED EXPOSURE FACTORS

400 RS, small focus, 100 mA, 0.05 sec, 60 kVp, 40″ SID, nongrid

PROCEDURES

1. Visually inspect the cassette and screens. Give particular attention to the following:

   a. Loose, worn, or broken hinges and catches
   b. Locking straps or catches that are not holding securely
   c. Warped, twisted, or cracked frames
   d. Frayed or excessively worn or loose felt
   e. Screens improperly installed in the cassette
   f. Dust, dirt, scratches, chips, or stains on the screens
   g. Deterioration of the screen's protective layer

2. If the screens appear dirty or if they have not been cleaned recently, proceed as follows:

   a. Use screen cleaner solution or a mild soap and water solution to dampen a clean gauze sponge.

   b. Wipe one screen at a time with the gauze sponge in vertical lines, then repeat the process horizontally. After cleaning, wipe each screen with a dry gauze sponge.

   c. Leave cassettes open until the screens are thoroughly dry.

   d. Record the date on the appropriate label on the rear of the cassette; if none exists, fashion one out of tape and fasten it to the cassette with the necessary information recorded.

   e. If a screen cleaning log is kept, record the cassette number and date cleaned in the appropriate place.

LABORATORY 33-8 (Continued)

3. Load a clean cassette with fresh film. Wait 5 minutes to ensure that any trapped air has escaped.

4. Place the cassette in the center of the radiographic table, center the tube to the cassette and collimate to the cassette size using a 40″ SID.

5. Place the wire mesh test tool on top of the cassette. Expose the cassette using suggested exposure factors.

6. Process the film. A density of 1.2 to 1.5 should be obtained to make a proper evaluation. If necessary, repeat this step until the appropriate density is achieved.

RESULTS

1. Place the test image on a radiographic illuminator in a dimly lit environment.

2. View the image at a distance of 6 to 9 feet.

3. Areas of poor film/screen contact will be demonstrated by areas of increased density or nonuniformity of density and a cloudy or hazy appearance.

4. Areas of poor contact that exist around the perimeter of the cassette may be considered acceptable provided they do not extend more than 1 inch into the film. Areas of poor contact in the center of the image are completely unacceptable.

5. For new cassettes the previous criteria should be more rigid than for older cassettes.

ANALYSIS

1. Did the cassettes tested pass the film/screen contact test? If not, describe the appearance of the images.

2. What is the clinical importance of film/screen contact?

3. Give at least two reasons why it is essential to maintain screen cleanliness.

LABORATORY 33-9 EVALUATING VIEW BOX UNIFORMITY

PURPOSE

Evaluate the uniformity of radiographic view boxes (illuminators).

FOR FURTHER REVIEW

Refer to Chapter 33 in the accompanying textbook for further review of this topic.

MATERIALS

1. Light meter

2. Test mask (14″ × 17″ cardboard with a hole cut in the center of each of four quadrants)

3. View boxes, at least two separate banks of multiple panels

PROCEDURES

1. Clean any dirty view boxes, including inside, with a wet cloth.

2. Place the test mask on the view box to be evaluated. The mask is divided into four quadrants, each containing a hole for the light meter.

3. Position the light meter over the upper left quadrant and record the reading. Illumination (intensity) level can be measured as lux, foot-candle (fc), or exposure value (eV), depending on the type of light meter being used.

4. Repeat step 3 for the other quadrants and record the readings.

5. Repeat Procedures 1 through 4 for all other view box panels to be tested and record the appropriate data. Most view box panels are grouped together to form a bank. With this in mind it is sensible to test the variation of illumination level between the panels, which together form a bank. Since these banks of view boxes will be found in different areas around the radiology department, it is also wise to test the variation in illumination levels between the separate banks of view boxes.

6. Record the room (ambient) light level for the viewing area.

7. Using the recorded test results, calculate and record the following:

   a. Determine the average illumination level for each view box panel.

   $$\text{Avg. } I_P = (I_{q1} + I_{q2} + I_{q3} + I_{q4}) \div 4$$

   b. Determine the average illumination level for the entire bank of view box panels.

   $$\text{Avg. } I_B = (\text{Avg. } I_{P1} + \text{Avg. } I_{P2} + \text{..........} \text{ Avg. } I_{pn}) \div n$$

   c. For each view box panel, determine the maximum variation in the illumination level between quadrants.

   $$V_{IP} = (I_{q\,max} - I_{q\,min}) / (I_{q\,max} + I_{q\,min}) \times 100\%$$

d. Determine the maximum variation between the averages of the individual panels for a given bank of view boxes.

$$V_{IB} = (\text{Avg. } I_{p\,max} - \text{Avg. } I_{p\,min}) / (\text{Avg. } I_{p\,max} + \text{Avg. } I_{p\,min}) \times 100 \text{ percent}$$

e. Determine the maximum variation between the averages of different view box banks within a radiology department.

$$V_{IG} = (\text{Avg. } I_{B\,max} - \text{Avg. } I_{B\,min}) / (\text{Avg. } I_{B\,max} + \text{Avg. } I_{B\,min}) \times 100 \text{ percent}$$

RESULTS

VIEW BOX BANK _____

Panel	I_{q1}	I_{q2}	I_{q3}	I_{q4}	Avg. I_P	V_{IP}

Avg. I_B = _____ V_{IB} = _____   Ambient Light Level _____

Acceptance Criteria

View box illumination level: minimum of 500 fc or 13 eV at 100 ASA
Ambient room light level: maximum of 8 fc or 8 eV at 100 ASA

$V_{IP} \leq 10$ percent $V_{IB} \leq 15$ percent $V_{IG} \leq 20$ percent

ANALYSIS

1. Did the ambient light level(s) for the view box(es) tested pass the acceptance criteria? If not, what was the percent error?

2. What effect might an overly bright reading area have on viewing an image?

3. Did all the view box panels tested pass the acceptance criteria for illumination level and uniformity? If not, which ones were not acceptable and what was the percent error?

4. What effect might a dim view box have on viewing an image?

5. What effect might the lack of illumination uniformity of a view box have on viewing an image?

6. Did all the banks of view boxes tested pass the acceptance criteria for illumination uniformity between the panels? If not, which ones were not acceptable and what was the percent error?

7. What effect might the lack of illumination uniformity between panels on a bank of view boxes have on viewing images?

8. If separate banks of view boxes were tested, did they pass the acceptance criteria for illumination uniformity? If not, which ones were not acceptable and what was the percent error?

9. What effect might the lack of illumination uniformity between banks of view boxes have on viewing images?

10. Describe at least four possible causes for illumination problems associated with view boxes.

LABORATORY 33-10 REPEAT IMAGE STUDIES

PURPOSE

Analyze repeated images in a radiology department.

FOR FURTHER REVIEW

Refer to Chapter 33 in the accompanying textbook for further review of this topic.

MATERIALS

1. Images repeated during a survey period

2. Repeat analysis worksheet

PROCEDURES

1. Establish a method to accurately determine the amount of film used (i.e., record films, multiply average films per exam by number of exams recorded, computerized film usage, etc.).

2. Set a start date and length for the survey period. Clean out all repeat film bins to begin the study. (A 4-week survey period is recommended.)

3. At the end of the survey period collect all repeated images and determine the total number of images used during this period.

4. Analyze the repeated images to determine the reason that they were probably repeated, using the categories listed on the repeat analysis worksheet.

RESULTS

1. Using the repeat analysis worksheet, record the number of repeated images in each repeat category against the exam type they represent according to the exam categories listed on the next page.

ANALYSIS

1. Calculate the monthly repeat rate (%) based on the data collected for the survey period.

2. Calculate the repeat rate (%) of repeated images by repeat reason category.

3. Calculate the repeat rate (%) of repeated images by exam category.

4. List suggestions for corrective measures (actions) to minimize the repeat rates in the problem areas identified.

LABORATORY 33-10 (Continued)

REPEAT ANALYSIS WORKSHEET

SURVEY PERIOD _____ to _____ LOCATION _____

Repeat Category Exam	Position	Over-exposed	Under-exposed	Motion	Artifacts	Other	Total	%
Chest								
Ribs								
Shoulder								
Humerus								
Elbow								
Forearm								
Wrist								
Hand								
C–Spine								
T–Spine								
L–Spine								
Skull								
Facial								
Sinuses								
Abdomen								
Pelvis								
Hip								
Femur								
Knee								
Lower Leg								
Ankle								
Foot								
UGI								
LGI								
IVP								
Other								
TOTAL								
%								

LABORATORY 33-11 DARKROOM SAFELIGHT TEST

PURPOSE

Evaluate the safelight conditions and the sensitivity of exposed and unexposed radiographic film to a darkroom safelight.

FOR FURTHER REVIEW

Refer to Chapter 33 in the accompanying textbook for further review of this topic.

MATERIALS

1. Energized radiographic unit

2. Film processor

3. 10″ × 12″ cassette and image receptor

4. 10″ × 12″ piece of cardboard

5. Densitometer

SUGGESTED EXPOSURE FACTORS

400 RS, 25 mA, 0.017 sec, 40 kVp, 40″ SID, nongrid

PROCEDURES

1. Mask the cassette in half, center to the unmasked area, collimate, and expose the film. Remove the film from the cassette in the darkroom in total darkness and lay it on the darkroom countertop.

2. Place a piece of cardboard crosswise over the entire film, leaving approximately 1 inch at the top. Place a small pencil mark on the edge of the film where the cardboard cover was placed. Turn on all of the safelights normally used in the darkroom.

3. Expose the first 1-inch strip for 1 minute to the safelight illumination. Following the first exposure, slide the cardboard down approximately 1 additional inch, mark the film edge and expose for another minute. Expose five successive 1-inch sections at 1-minute intervals, following the same procedure. Leave a 1-inch strip on the bottom unexposed to any safelight. This procedure produces strips of the film with 0 through 3 minutes of safelight exposure.

4. Turn off all safelights and process the film.

5. Record the densitometer readings on both halves of all the 1-inch sections of the test film. When the film is processed, the exposed side should yield a density in the 0.35 to 1.0 density range. The film is unacceptable if the density is not within this range and the procedure should be repeated with an appropriate adjustment of exposure factors.

RESULTS

Time Exposed to Safelight	Optical Density Exposed Half	Unexposed Half
3 minutes	_____	_____
2 minutes	_____	_____
1 minutes	_____	_____
0 minutes	_____	_____

Acceptance Criteria

The difference between the exposed side and the unexposed side should be ≤ 0.02 OD.

ANALYSIS

1. Describe the effects of safelight illumination on radiographic density. Did the results of the safelight test pass the acceptance criteria? How close do the densitometric results agree with your visual observations?

2. Did the exposed and nonexposed sides of the film respond equally to the test? If different, how?

3. Based on your results, would you estimate that film in the film bin or an exposed film would be more sensitive to darkroom safelight fog? If different, what do you believe would cause the difference?

4. How could you determine whether the fog received was due to safelights or to light leaks around openings?

5. What is the safelight filter type used in the experiment? List the bulb wattage and approximate distance from the film for the safelight(s) used.

UNIT V   Comparing Exposure Systems

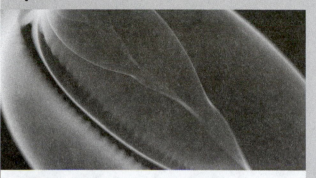

WORKSHEET 34–1 COMPARING EXPOSURE SYSTEMS

PURPOSE
Compare various types of exposure systems.

FOR FURTHER REVIEW
Refer to Chapter 34 in the accompanying textbook for further review of this topic.

ACTIVITIES

Answer the following questions:

  1. What is the goal of a radiographic exposure system?

  2. How do radiographic exposure systems function (generically) to achieve this goal?

  3. Describe a fixed optimum kilovoltage exposure system.

  4. List at least three advantages and three disadvantages associated with this type of system.

  5. Describe a variable kilovoltage exposure system.

  6. List at least three advantages and three disadvantages associated with this type of system.

  7. Describe an automatic exposure control (AEC) exposure system.

  8. List at least three advantages and three disadvantages associated with this type of system.

9. Fill in the missing steps in the establishment of a technique chart.

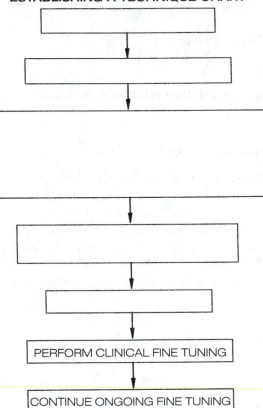

ESTABLISHING A TECHNIQUE CHART

PERFORM CLINICAL FINE TUNING

CONTINUE ONGOING FINE TUNING

WORKSHEET 34-2 ESTABLISHING A TECHNIQUE CHART

PURPOSE

Establish a technique chart.

FOR FURTHER REVIEW

Refer to Chapter 34 in the accompanying textbook for further review of this topic.

ACTIVITIES

Use the following scenarios to answer the following questions.

Scenario 1. A newly constructed orthopedic clinic has hired you to run one radiology room. The radiographic unit is a 500 mA three-phase, six-pulse generator and is not equipped with automatic exposure control. A rare-earth image receptor system is being used. One of your initial duties will be to establish a technique chart to be used in the facility. The manager of the clinic is willing to provide you with any of the resources that you will need to accomplish this task.

1. What type of exposure system are you going to use in developing your technique chart? Justify your decision.

2. You will begin the production of your technique chart by developing techniques for a lumbar spine. Describe the steps you would take to establish a reliable technique chart for lumbar spine examinations.

Scenario 2. You are responsible for a quality control program in a 10-room radiology department in a 400-bed community hospital. The department includes four general radiographic rooms, one dedicated chest unit, three digital fluoroscopic rooms, a digital vascular/interventional room, and one emergency radiographic room with a table and upright bucky device. All generators are high frequency and equipped with AEC except for one general radiographic room, which has a three-phase, six-pulse generator and no AEC. A 400 RS rare-earth imaging system is currently being used. You have been charged with developing a technique system to be used in the facility. The department head is willing to provide you with any of the resources that you will need to accomplish this task.

3. What type of exposure system will you use to develop your technique chart? Justify your decision.

4. Describe the steps you would take to establish a reliable technique system for use in the general diagnostic area.

5. After developing technique charts for the general diagnostic area, how would you go about designing a technique chart for use in the ER suite?

LABORATORY 35-1 DEVELOPING A FIXED kVp TECHNIQUE CHART

PURPOSE

Construct a fixed kVp technique chart.

FOR FURTHER REVIEW

Refer to Chapters 34 and 35 in the accompanying textbook for further review of this topic.

MATERIALS

1. Energized radiographic unit

2. Automatic film processor

3. Abdomen phantom

4. 14″ × 17″ radiographic cassettes with image receptor

PROCEDURES

1. Position the abdomen phantom for an AP projection and measure its thickness at the CR entrance point.

2. Determine appropriate technical factors for a diagnostic quality image receptor exposure, expose, and process a film.

3. Evaluate the quality of the image. Repeat step 2 until a satisfactory diagnostic quality image receptor exposure is achieved. Record the exposure factors used on all images along with the words "fixed kVp."

4. Produce four more images of the phantom using two different kVp levels above and two different kVp levels below the kVp used on the first image. Use the 15 percent rule or any other technique compensation system to adjust the mAs to compensate for the kVp changes. Repeat the images until all four images display the same radiographic receptor exposure as the first one.

5. Review all five of the test images and eliminate the ones that you believe are unacceptable. Of the images remaining, the one with the highest kVp will be considered the optimal image. Write "optimal image" on this image. The kVp used to produce the "optimal image" is the fixed optimal kVp for that body part.

6. Complete the fixed kVp technique chart in the Results section by extrapolating the required mAs values for the different part thickness based on the mAs used to obtain the optimal image.

LABORATORY 35-1 (Continued)

RESULTS

FIXED kVp TECHNIQUE CHART

PART _____

PROJECTION _____

_____ kVp

_____ " SID

_____ Relative Speed

_____ Tabletop

_____ Grid/Bucky

_____ Grid Ratio

COMMENTS:

cm	mAs
16	
17	
18	
19	
20	
21	
22	
23	
24	
25	
26	
27	
28	
29	
30	
31	
32	
33	

ANALYSIS

1. Based on your experience in this laboratory, discuss the fixed kVp approach to technique development with respect to accuracy, quality of results, ease of use, and usefulness in modifying established techniques.

2. Based on your experience, discuss the advantages and disadvantages of using the fixed kVp system in a clinical situation.

LABORATORY 36-1 DEVELOPING A VARIABLE kVp TECHNIQUE CHART

PURPOSE

Construct a variable kVp technique chart.

FOR FURTHER REVIEW

Refer to Chapters 35 and 36 in the accompanying textbook for further review of this topic.

MATERIALS

1. Energized radiographic unit

2. Automatic film processor

3. Abdomen phantom

4. 14″ × 17″ radiographic cassettes with image receptor

PROCEDURES

1. Position the abdomen phantom for an AP projection and measure its thickness at the central ray entrance point.

2. Determine the kVp to be used according to the (cm × 2) + 30 kVp formula. Choose an mAs value, based on the body part, part thickness, kVp, and SID that you feel will produce a diagnostic quality image. Expose and process a film.

3. Evaluate the quality of the image. Repeat step 2 until a satisfactory diagnostic quality image is achieved. Record the exposure factors used on all images and label them "standard variable kVp."

4. Produce four more images of the phantom using two different kVp levels above and two different kVp levels below the kVp used on the first image. Use the 15 percent rule or any other technique compensation system to adjust the mAs to compensate for the kVp changes. Repeat the films until all four images display the same radiographic receptor exposure as the first one.

5. Review all five of the test images and eliminate the ones that you believe unacceptable (pay particular attention to the contrast). Of the images remaining, the one with the highest kVp will be considered the low-contrast limit and the one with the lowest kVp will be considered the high-contrast limit. All the images between these limits would presumably have acceptable contrast, assuming the radiographic exposure is adequate. Record the kVp values that represent the chosen limits.

6. Complete the variable kVp technique chart in the Results section by extrapolating the required kVp values for the different part thickness based on a 2 kVp change per cm thickness. During the extrapolation when the kVp reaches either the low- or high-contrast limit recorded earlier, adjust the kVp (with the appropriate mAs compensation) to bring it back to the beginning of the acceptable contrast range. Then continue the extrapolation.

LABORATORY 36-1 (Continued)

RESULTS

FIXED kVp TECHNIQUE CHART

PART _____

PROJECTION _____

_____   " SID

_____   Relative Speed

_____   Tabletop

_____   Grid/Bucky

_____   Grid Ratio

COMMENTS:

cm	kVp	mAs
16		
17		
18		
19		
20		
21		
22		
23		
24		
25		
26		
27		
28		
29		
30		
31		
32		
33		

ANALYSIS

1. Based on your experience in this laboratory, discuss the variable kVp approach to technique development with respect to accuracy, quality of results, ease of use, and usefulness in modifying established techniques.

2. Based on your experience, discuss the advantages and disadvantages of using the variable kVp system in a clinical situation.

LABORATORY 37-1 DETERMINING AND CONTROLLING ION CHAMBER CONFIGURATIONS

PURPOSE

Demonstrate the configuration and correct selection of ion chambers in an automatic exposure control device.

FOR FURTHER REVIEW

Refer to Chapter 37 in the accompanying textbook for further review of this topic.

MATERIALS

1. Energized radiographic unit equipped with ion chamber automatic exposure control
2. Automatic film processor
3. 14″ × 17″ cassette with film matched to AEC system being tested
4. Abdomen or pelvis phantom

SUGGESTED EXPOSURE FACTORS

400 RS, 100 mA, phototimed, 80 kVp, 40″ SID, 8:1 Bucky grid

PROCEDURES

1. Set the tube to 40″ SID, center to the table, place a loaded 14″ × 17″ cassette in the Bucky tray, align to the central ray, and collimate the beam to the film size.

2. Set the generator for manual technique control (deactivate the automatic exposure device [phototimer]), expose, and process the film.

3. Evaluate the image carefully to see if the location of the ion chambers can be visualized (faintly). Repeat the film with appropriate mAs adjustments if necessary.

4. Set the tube to 40″ SID, center to the table, position the phantom for an AP projection, place a loaded 14″ × 17″ cassette in the Bucky tray, align to the central ray, and collimate to the film size.

5. Select the normal density setting for the AEC system, use an mA station that is normally used with the AEC (usually 100 to 400 mA), use 80 kVp, select the center sensing chamber, expose, and process the film.

6. Produce another image by repeating steps 4 and 5 with one of the lateral sensing chambers selected.

7. Produce another image by repeating steps 4 and 5 with all three sensing chambers selected.

RESULTS

1. Review the first image and draw an arrow to the edges of each ion chamber.

2. Review the other images with respect to their radiographic exposure and image contrast.

LABORATORY 37-1 (Continued)

ANALYSIS

1. How many ion chambers were demonstrated on the first image? Are all the chambers of the same size?

2. Does the configuration of the chambers match the configuration demonstrated on the collimator template? If not or if there is no indication of chamber location on the collimator, describe the configuration in terms relevant to their use while positioning patients.

3. Describe the exposure and image contrast differences of the last three images.

4. Which image would be the most appropriate for an abdominal survey procedure? Why?

5. Which would be the most appropriate for a lumbar spine procedure? Why?

LABORATORY 37-2 THE EFFECT OF POSITIONING ON AUTOMATIC EXPOSURE CONTROL

PURPOSE

Demonstrate the effect of positioning errors on the image quality of automatic exposure control radiographs.

FOR FURTHER REVIEW

Refer to Chapter 37 in the accompanying textbook for further review of this topic.

MATERIALS

1. Energized radiographic unit with automatic exposure control

2. Automatic film processor

3. 14″ × 17″ cassette with film matched to AEC system being tested

4. Abdomen or pelvis phantom

SUGGESTED EXPOSURE FACTORS

400 RS, 400 mA, phototimed, 80 kVp, 40″ SID, 8:1 Bucky grid

PROCEDURES

1. Set the tube to a 40″ SID, center to the table, position the phantom for a lateral lumbar spine, place a loaded 14″ × 17″ cassette in the Bucky tray, align to the central ray, and collimate to the spine (approximately 6″ × 17″).

2. Select the normal density setting for the AEC system, use an mA station that is normally used with the AEC (usually 100 to 400 mA), use 80 kVp, select the center chamber, expose, and process the film.

3. Produce a second image by repeating steps 1 and 2 with the phantom moved 1.5″ posteriorly.

4. Produce a third image by repeating steps 1 and 2 with the phantom moved 1.5″ anteriorly.

RESULTS

1. Review the three images with respect to radiographic exposure and image contrast.

ANALYSIS

1. Which image exhibits the best exposure quality? Why?

2. Which image exhibits the worst exposure quality? Why?

3. What caused the exposure quality to change between the first and second images?

4. What caused the exposure quality to change between the first and third images?

LABORATORY 37-3 THE EFFECT OF COLLIMATION ON AUTOMATIC EXPOSURE CONTROL

PURPOSE

Demonstrate the effects and control of scatter radiation on automatic exposure control radiographs.

FOR FURTHER REVIEW

Refer to Chapter 37 in the accompanying textbook for further review of this topic.

MATERIALS

1. Energized radiographic unit equipped with automatic exposure control

2. Automatic film processor

3. 14″ × 17″ cassette with film matched to the AEC system being tested

4. Abdomen or pelvis phantom

5. Lead masks

SUGGESTED EXPOSURE FACTORS

400 RS, 400 mA, phototimed, 80 kVp, 40″ SID, 8:1 Bucky grid

PROCEDURES

1. Set the tube to a 40″ SID, center to the table, position the phantom for a lateral lumbar spine, place a loaded 14″ × 17″ cassette in the Bucky tray, align to the central ray, and collimate to the film size.

2. Select the normal density setting for the AEC system, use an mA station that is normally used with the AEC (usually 100 to 400 mA), use 80 kVp, select the center ion chamber, expose, and process the film.

3. Produce a second image by repeating steps 1 and 2 with the beam collimated to the lumbar spine (6″ × 17″).

4. Produce a third image by repeating steps 1 and 2 with the beam collimated to the lumbar spine (6″ × 17″) with the addition of lead masks on the table to outline the posterior aspect of the soft tissue. Position the lead masks carefully so as not to overlap the posterior aspect of the phantom.

RESULTS

1. Review the three images with respect to radiographic exposure and image contrast.

ANALYSIS

1. Which image exhibits the best exposure quality? Why?

2. Which image exhibits the worst exposure quality? Why?

3. What caused the image exposure to change between the first and second images?

4. What caused the image exposure to change between the second and third images?

LABORATORY 37-4 EVALUATING AUTOMATIC EXPOSURE CONTROLS

PURPOSE

Evaluate the performance of automatic exposure control kVp compensation and response capability.

FOR FURTHER REVIEW

Refer to Chapter 37 in the accompanying textbook for further review of this topic.

MATERIALS

1. Energized radiographic unit with automatic exposure control

2. Automatic film processor

3. Two aluminum (1100 alloy) plates 7″ × 7″ × 3/4″

4. One cassette with film matched to the AEC system being tested

5. Densitometer

6. Lead identification markers

SUGGESTED EXPOSURE FACTORS

See procedure.

PROCEDURES

1. Set the tube to a 40″ SID, center to the table, position one Al plate to the center of the light field, and collimate the field to slightly less than the dimensions of the aluminum plate. Place the lead markers along the edge of the field to label the film #1.

2. Place a loaded cassette in the Bucky tray, align to the central ray, select the normal density setting for the AEC system, use an mA station that is normally used with the AEC (usually 100 to 400 mA), use 70 kVp, select the center chamber, expose, and process the film.

3. Using the same cassette, repeat steps 1 and 2, label the image #2, but use 85 kVp. Repeat the procedure again labeling the image #3 and using 100 kVp.

4. Place the second Al plate on top of the first and repeat procedures 1 through 3, labeling the images #3, 4, and 5.

RESULTS

1. Measure the optical exposures of the six images in the center of each image with a densitometer and record the following readings as a function of kVp versus thickness of aluminum.

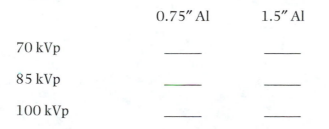

	0.75″ Al	1.5″ Al
70 kVp	_____	_____
85 kVp	_____	_____
100 kVp	_____	_____

LABORATORY 37-4 (Continued)

2. Evaluate the test data against an acceptance criterion of $\pm$ OD 0.20 for the kVp compensation and response capability tests.

ANALYSIS

1. Do your test results meet the acceptance criteria for the parameters tested?

2. What might be some possible problems with the AEC device that would cause the densities to exceed the acceptance criteria for these tests?

3. What is meant by the minimum response time of an AEC system?

4. What is the purpose of the backup timer in an AEC system?

5. It has been suggested that a fixed kVp exposure technique system be used with AEC devices when using rare-earth imaging systems. Defend this statement.

WORKSHEET 38-1 SOLVING MULTIPLE EFFECTS PROBLEMS

PURPOSE

Practice solving multiple effect exposure problems.

FOR FURTHER REVIEW

Refer to Chapter 38 in the accompanying textbook for further review of this topic.

ACTIVITIES

Select the set of exposure factors that would produce the greatest image receptor exposure for questions 1 through 7.

		mA	Time	kVp	SID	Screens (Relative Speed)	Grid
1.	(a)	100	1/5 sec	65			
	(b)	200	1/10 sec	70			
	(c)	50	2/5 sec	65			
	(d)	400	1/20 sec	60			
2.	(a)	300	0.04 sec		40"		
	(b)	600	0.025 sec		36"		
	(c)	800	0.015 sec		40"		
	(d)	200	0.05 sec		36"		
3.	(a)	100	1/10 sec	68	36"		
	(b)	75	1/5 sec	68	36"		
	(c)	400	1/20 sec	68	36"		
	(d)	600	1/60 sec	68	36"		
4.	(a)	500	0.02 sec	80		100	
	(b)	1000	0.01 sec	75		100	
	(c)	300	0.05 sec	80		100	
	(d)	600	0.033 sec	75		100	
5.	(a)	500	1/5 sec				8:1
	(b)	1000	1/10 sec				12:1
	(c)	1000	1/8 sec				8:1
	(d)	500	1/4 sec				12:1
6.	(a)	400	150 msec	75	36"	200	12:1
	(b)	500	80 msec	75	36"	200	16:1
	(c)	800	150 msec	75	36"	200	12:1
	(d)	1500	20 msec	75	36"	200	8:1
7.	(a)	200	1/20 sec	65	40"	100	8:1
	(b)	150	1/10 sec	60	50"	100	8:1
	(c)	300	1/30 sec	65	50"	100	8:1
	(d)	200	1/10 sec	60	60"	100	8:1

8. A satisfactory image is produced using a single-phase, fully rectified generator, 75 kVp, 200 mA, 0.10 sec, 40″ SID, 400 RS, and an 8:1 grid. What exposure time would be required to produce a new image with the same image receptor exposure if a three-phase, 12-pulse generator, 100 mA, 100 RS, and 5:1 grid are used?

9. A satisfactory image is produced using a three-phase, 12-pulse generator, 60 kVp, 6.6 mAs, 36″ SID, 100 RS, without a grid. What mAs would be required to produce a new image with the same image receptor exposure if a three-phase, six-pulse generator, 65 kVp, 40″ SID, 400 RS, and an 8:1 grid are used?

10. A satisfactory image is produced for a 20 cm AP pelvis using a three-phase,12-pulse generator, 80 kVp, 30 mAs, 40″ SID, 300 RS, and a 12:1 grid. What mAs would be required to produce a new image with the same image receptor exposure for a 24 cm AP pelvis if a single-phase, two-pulse generator, 92 kVp, 60″ SID, 800 RS, and 5:1 grid are used?

Special Imaging Systems

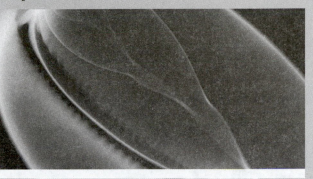

LABORATORY 39-1 THE EFFECT OF ALIGNMENT AND DISTANCE ON MOBILE RADIOGRAPHIC IMAGE QUALITY

PURPOSE

Demonstrate the effect of central ray alignment and distance on image quality during mobile procedures.

FOR FURTHER REVIEW

Refer to Chapter 39 in the accompanying textbook for further review of this topic.

MATERIALS

1. Energized radiographic unit

2. Automatic film processor

3. 10″ × 12″ cassette with image receptor

4. Coconut (milk-filled) (when buying coconut, shake to hear milk)

SUGGESTED EXPOSURE FACTORS

400 RS, 100 mA, 0.05 sec, 5 mAs, 50 kVp, 40″ SID

PROCEDURES

Alignment Problems

1. Place the coconut in the center of a 10″ × 12″ cassette, direct the central ray to the center of the cassette, collimate to the film size, set the tube to a 40″ SID, label the film #1, expose, and process the film.

2. Place the cassette in a vertical position, label the film #2, and use a horizontal beam to repeat step 1 (use sponges as necessary to place the coconut in the center of the film).

3. Place the cassette on a 45° angle to the plane of the floor, label the film #3, and use a horizontal beam to repeat step 1.

4. Place the cassette on a 45° angle to the plane of the floor, label the film #4, direct the central ray perpendicular to the film, and repeat step 1.

Estimating Distance

1. Conceal the distance indicator on the radiographic unit, estimate a 36″ SID, then reveal the distance indicator and record the actual SID.

2. Repeat step 1 estimating 40″, 56″, and 72″ SIDs.

Distance/Density Problems

1. Place the coconut in the center of a 10″ × 12″ cassette, direct the central ray to the center of the cassette, collimate to the film size, set the tube to a 36″ SID, label the film #5, expose, and process the film.

2. Repeat step 1, using a 38″ SID for film #6, a 40″ SID for film #7, and a 42″ SID for film #8.

RESULTS

Estimating Distance

1. Record the actual distance for the following estimated distances:

   36" SID _____

   40" SID _____

   56" SID _____

   72" SID _____

ANALYSIS

Alignment Problems

1. Review images #1 through 4. Which of the images demonstrate a sharp air-fluid level within the coconut?

2. What is the proper procedure to demonstrate air-fluid levels in a patient?

3. What effects do image receptor and tube placement have on the demonstration of air-fluid levels?

Estimating Distance

4. How close were the actual distances to the estimated distances?

5. What effect will estimating distance for a mobile procedure have on image quality?

Distance/Density Problems

6. Review films #5 through 8. What effects do small changes in distance have on radiographic exposure?

7. How much of a distance change is necessary to notice the effect of the change on the image?

LABORATORY 40-1 OPERATING FLUOROSCOPIC SPOT FILMING SYSTEMS

PURPOSE

Operate a fluoroscopic spot filming system.

FOR FURTHER REVIEW

Refer to Chapter 40 in the accompanying textbook for further review of this topic.

MATERIALS

1. Energized fluoroscopic unit

2. Lead apron

3. Spot film camera or spot film cassettes

4. Large radiographic phantom (e.g., chest, abdomen, or pelvis)

5. Automatic film processor

EXPOSURE FACTORS

Suggested Factors

Medium mA (by setting brightness control) at 70 to 120 kVp

PROCEDURES

1. Wearing a lead apron, place the phantom at the center of the fluoroscopic unit and move the carriage into the operating position.

2. Use the foot pedal to turn the fluoroscope on. Move the carriage until the phantom is centered to the image.

3. Use the carriage controls to set the spot film system to a 4-on-1 position and make two spot film exposures. Move the carriage slightly and then set the spot film system to a 2-on-1 position so that a single exposure will completely fill the remaining portion of the film. Make the exposure and process the film.

RESULTS

1. Mark the film to show which exposure was made first, second, and third.

ANALYSIS

1. Draw each of the possible spot film exposure configurations available on the fluoroscopic unit that was used.

2. Describe at least one clinical examination for which each of the following spot film configurations would be most useful: 4-on-1, 2-on-1 vertical, 2-on-1 horizontal, and 1-on-1.

LABORATORY 40-2 FLUOROSCOPIC AUTOMATIC BRIGHTNESS CONTROLS

PURPOSE

Explain the basic function of a fluoroscopic automatic brightness control.

FOR FURTHER REVIEW

Refer to Chapter 40 in the accompanying textbook for further review of this topic.

MATERIALS

1. Energized fluoroscopic unit

2. Lead apron

3. Spot film camera or spot film cassettes

4. Large radiographic phantom (e.g., chest, abdomen, or pelvis)

5. Automatic film processor

EXPOSURE FACTORS

Suggested Factors

Medium mA (by setting brightness control) at 70 to 120 kVp

PROCEDURES

1. Wearing a lead apron, place the phantom at the center of the fluoroscopic unit and move the carriage into the operating position.

2. Use the foot pedal to turn the fluoroscope on. Move the carriage until the phantom is centered to the image.

3. Move the carriage slowly from the center of the phantom to one side, observing the image closely during the motion.

4. Return the carriage slowly to the center of the phantom and then move it gradually up or down until the phantom disappears from the image.

ANALYSIS

1. Describe how the image changes as the fluoroscope moves from a thick portion of the phantom to a thin region.

2. Explain the mechanism that causes the changes described in #1.

WORKSHEET 41–1 RADIOGRAPHIC TOMOGRAPHY

PURPOSE

Explain the differences between diagnostic radiographic equipment and equipment specialized for radiographic tomography.

FOR FURTHER REVIEW

Refer to Chapter 41 in the accompanying textbook for further review of this topic.

ACTIVITIES

1. Explain the basis for radiographic tomography.

2. Define *tomographic amplitude* and describe its relationship to the tomographic section thickness.

3. Define *fulcrum* and describe its relationship to the focal plane.

4. What types of motion are employed in radiographic tomography?

5. How do changes in the tomographic motion affect the tomographic image?

6. Which exposure factor is most critical when performing radiographic tomography? Why?

7. What are the most common uses of radiographic tomography in a modern imaging department?

LABORATORY 41-2 RADIOGRAPHIC TOMOGRAPHY MOTION

PURPOSE

Determine the path of the x-ray beam during a radiographic tomography exposure.

FOR FURTHER REVIEW

Refer to Chapter 41 in the accompanying textbook for further review of this topic.

MATERIALS

1. Energized tomographic unit

2. Automatic film processor

3. 8″ × 10″ cassette with film

4. Tomographic phantom (commercial or homemade), typically consisting of a number of acrylic discs. One disc contains lead numbers spaced 1 mm apart arranged in a helix so as to indicate slice level and thickness. One disc contains different size mesh pieces to evaluate focal plane resolution. Several discs of different thicknesses are to be used as spacers. The lead disc with a 4 mm aperture in the center evaluates beam uniformity and path.

SUGGESTED EXPOSURE FACTORS

200 RS, 60 mAs, 70 kVp, 40″ SID, 8:1 Bucky grid

PROCEDURES

1. Center the 4 cm spacer disc on the table, followed by the 1 cm and 2 cm spacers. Center the lead aperture disc on top of the stack of spacers.

2. Adjust the fulcrum of the system for 4.5 cm (45 mm).

3. Place the 8″ × 10″ cassette in the Bucky tray and collimate the beam to film size.

4. With the x-ray tube centered and perpendicular to the film, make a nontomographic exposure at the same kVp and about 10 percent of the mAs needed to properly expose the phantom. This exposure will mark the center of the pinhole trace.

5. Set the angle (arc) to the maximum routinely used. Make sure the exposure time is long enough to cover the complete tomographic arc and produce a tomographic exposure of the phantom.

6. Repeat the procedure in the opposite direction for linear tomographic equipment that exposes in both directions.

7. Process and evaluate the film. Depending on the phantom thickness, the pinhole trace may be too dark to interpret. An ideal density would be approximately 1.0, although it can vary greatly. A better exposure can be achieved by varying the number of spacers used. Repeat steps 1 through 7 if necessary to obtain an image.

LABORATORY 41-2 (Continued)

RESULTS

1. Review the test radiograph image for completeness and uniformity.
2. The image pattern represents the path of the beam during exposure.
3. The beam path should follow a smooth, uniform course. For linear tomography the beam path image should be equally divided on either side of the center (exposure) mark. Multidirectional units should not produce gaps or overlaps on the beam path image greater than 10 percent of the beam path length.
4. The optical density of the beam path image represents the uniformity of the exposure.
5. The density of the beam path should demonstrate minimal variations (less than 0.3 OD). Areas of increased and decreased density may indicate hesitation or changes in the speed of the tomographic sweep.

ANALYSIS

1. Does the image pattern of the tomographic phantom represent the tomographic motion used? Describe and explain.

2. Does the beam path image meet the criteria for completeness of motion? Describe and explain.

3. Does the uniformity of exposure appear to be acceptable? Describe and explain.

4. Explain the clinical importance of completeness and uniformity of tube motion during a tomographic study.

WORKSHEET 42-1 MAMMOGRAPHY EQUIPMENT

PURPOSE

Explain differences between diagnostic radiography equipment and that specialized for mammography.

FOR FURTHER REVIEW

Refer to Chapter 42 in the accompanying textbook for further review of this topic.

ACTIVITIES

1. What are the primary reasons for considering high-frequency generators for mammography?

2. What is the kVp range utilized in mammography?

3. Mammographic contrast must be sufficient to demonstrate microcalcifications that are extremely small. What is the size range that must be visualized adequately?

4. What is the major disadvantage of using kVp in the 20s range?

5. What is the typical mammography mA range?

6. What materials are used for the target of mammography x-ray tube anodes?

7. What is the minimum HVL required by the United States government for 30 kVp?

8. What is the range of mammography grid ratios and frequencies?

WORKSHEET 43–1 VASCULAR IMAGING EQUIPMENT

PURPOSE

Describe the imaging equipment used for specialized vascular and interventional radiologic procedures.

FOR FURTHER REVIEW

Refer to Chapter 43 in the accompanying textbook for further review of this topic.

ACTIVITIES

1. What are the three digital image acquisition modes used in vascular imaging? Explain the common uses for each mode.

2. What post-processing functions can be used to compensate for patient motion?

3. Why is a C-arm assembly commonly used in vascular imaging instead of a traditional fluoroscopic image intensification unit?

4. What are the five factors that affect injector flow rate?

WORKSHEET 44-1 COMPUTED TOMOGRAPHY

PURPOSE

Explain the basic features of computed tomographic units and the basic acquisition and display methods used in CT.

FOR FURTHER REVIEW

Refer to Chapter 44 in the accompanying textbook for further review of this topic.

ACTIVITIES

1. List the major characteristics of the first through the seventh generations of CT units.

2. What technology allows the use of helical scanning methods in CT?

3. Explain the term *multisection CT* and explain the significance of this development in CT scanning.

4. List the three parameters that determine detector dose efficiency.

5. Briefly explain how Hounsfield units are calculated and specify the HU associated with air, water, and bone.

6. What is a convolution filter?

7. Describe the relationship between the voxel, pixel, and matrix size in terms of image resolution.

8. What are the most common artifacts and their causes encountered in CT imaging?

9. List two parameters used to determine patient dose in computed tomographic imaging.

WORKSHEET 45-1 MAGNETIC RESONANCE IMAGING

PURPOSE

Explain the basic function of magnetic resonance imaging units, including the basic acquisition and display methods used in MRI.

FOR FURTHER REVIEW

Refer to Chapter 45 in the accompanying textbook for further review of this topic.

ACTIVITIES

1. What is the Larmor frequency and why is it critical to MR imaging?

2. Identify the primary parameters controlling the MRI process. Compare and contrast these parameters.

3. What purpose do gradient coils serve in acquiring an MR image? How many gradient coils are necessary to obtain an image and why?

4. What role do radio frequency pulse sequences play in obtaining various MR images?

5. What is the relationship between magnetic field strength and the images obtained in MR?

6. Highlight the key safety factors associated with magnetic resonance imaging.

7. Describe the differences in the image of a vertebral body on an MR and a CT image.

8. Describe the differences in the image of muscle on an MR and a CT image.

LABORATORY 45-2 EVALUATING MAGNETIC RESONANCE IMAGES

PURPOSE

Evaluate basic parameters of a magnetic resonance image.

FOR FURTHER REVIEW

Refer to Chapter 45 in the accompanying textbook for further review of this topic.

MATERIALS

1. Images from a complete abdominal magnetic resonance imaging examination with essentially normal anatomy imaged in transverse, sagittal, and coronal images

2. Images from a complete abdominal computed tomography examination with essentially normal anatomy (MRI and CT images may be from different patients)

ANALYSIS

1. Locate the following structures on transverse, sagittal, and coronal sections:

   a. vertebral body

   b. liver

   c. kidney

   d. aorta

   e. vena cava

2. Name an area that appears dark as a result of a signal void.

3. Describe the differences in the image of a vertebral body on the MR image with the CT image.

4. Describe the differences in the image of muscles on the MR image with the CT image.

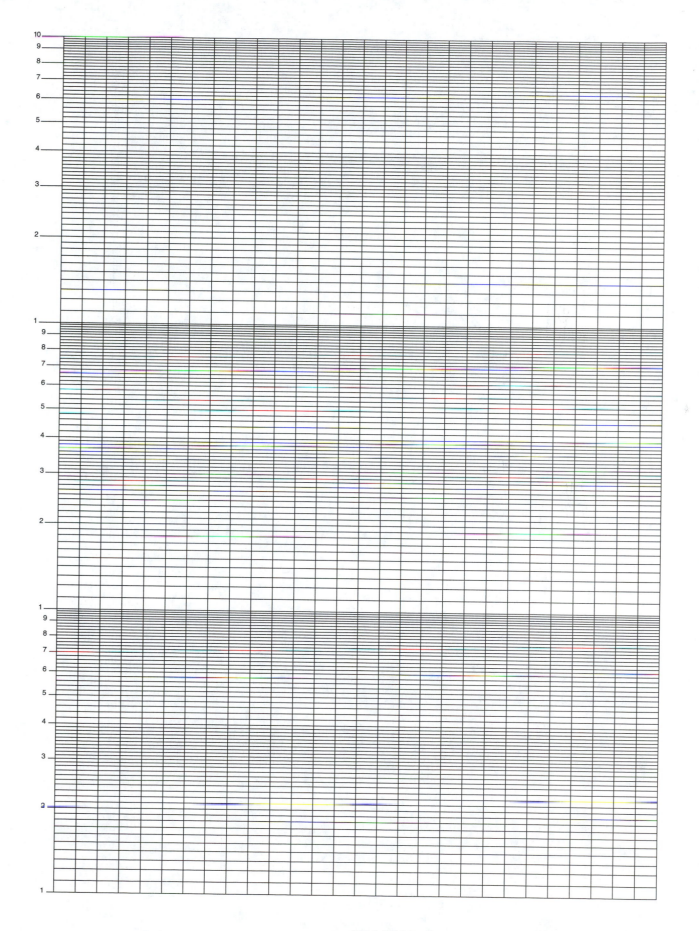